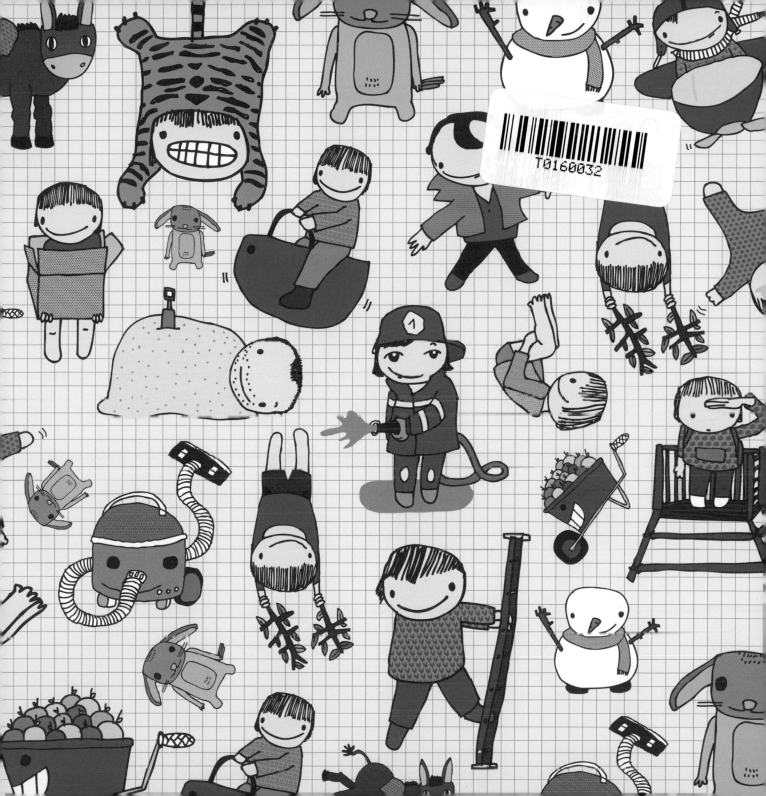

The authors, illustrator and publisher, or any other persons who have been involved in working on this publication, cannot accept responsiblity for any injuries or damage incurred as a result of the information or exercises contained in this book.
Please take care!

Rika Taeymans and Laura Van Bouchout
JACK'S ACROBATICS
A fun step-by-step guide to acrobatic exercise for the whole family

This first English language edition published by Pinter & Martin Ltd 2015

First published 2013 as *Nelsons Acrobatenboek* by Davidsfonds Uitgeverij nv, Belgium

Rika Taeymans and Laura Van Bouchout have asserted their moral rights to be identified as the authors of this work in accordance with the Copyright, Designs and Patents Act of 1988.

ISBN 978-1-78066-190-2

© 2013 Rika Taeymans, Laura Van Bouchout and Davidsfonds Uitgeverij nv
Foreword © 2015 Peter Duncan
Translated by Textcase

Illustration and design: Emma Thyssen
Cover design: Emma Thyssen

British Library Cataloguing-in-Publication Data
A catalogue record for this book is available from the British Library.

Printed in China by Everbest Printing Co. Ltd

Pinter & Martin Ltd
6 Effra Parade
London SW2 1PS

pinterandmartin.com

RIKA TAEYMANS & LAURA VAN BOUCHOUT
WITH ILLUSTRATIONS BY EMMA THYSSEN
FOREWORD PETER DUNCAN

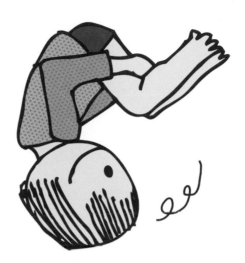

JACK'S ACROBATICS

A FUN STEP-BY-STEP GUIDE TO ACROBATIC EXERCISE FOR THE WHOLE FAMILY

pinter & martin

FOREWORD

One of my most vivid memories as a young child was when my father lay flat on his back with his arms outstretched above him – a challenge for me to stand on his hands. He would swing his legs up, I would grab them and then I would be 'flying'. I was performing what the writers of this wonderful book call The Lookout (see page 46). For me these early family romps were the spark that ignited an active and adventurous life.

The laughter, gasps and contact between grown-up and child has benefits that dispel the more passive pursuits of our digital age. We are, after all, apes and *Jack's Acrobatics* inspires us to balance, twist and tumble in a way many of our species have forgotten how to do.

Every young person should be a Jack and every parent a stable bridge so our imaginative minds and clever bodies are in harmony.

Do it now. Are you ready? Hup... hup... ho!

Peter Duncan
actor, TV presenter and documentary maker
former BBC *Blue Peter* presenter and UK Chief Scout
heresoneimadeearlier.com

TO BEGIN WITH...

Pure pleasure. *Jack's Acrobatics* sprouted from this core principle. For twenty years, I've been getting up very early every Saturday morning to give more than a hundred children lessons in 'circomotorics' with their mum or dad. Every week, I see children blossom through developmental movement games and acrobatic exercises, dads laughing and mums enjoying horsing around with their children.

Our busy lives often prevent us from fully interacting with our children. Physical contact, however, is as important to them as the air they breathe. Playing together works wonders not only for the development of your child, but for the relationship between you and your child as well.

Jack's Acrobatics provides a means by which you can deepen the bond between you and your child through challenging motor-skill games and with the use of play. The most important criterion of this book is to have fun together. The hope is for you and your child to thoroughly enjoy yourselves – just like Jack.

STEP BY STEP

It's your child, and not Jack, who sets the pace in this book. *Jack's Acrobatics* aims to provide you and your child with successes that are attainable for you both. By means of simple practice games, Jack's step-by-step guide helps you to develop acrobatics skills. This structure was chosen purposely – without preparatory exercises, children are more prone to give up.

You can rest at anytime. There's no point in forcing things. In my own classes, I start and finish every exercise in the rocking chair (see page 52). This exercise offers kids a clear structure and the chance to rest. At times, you might only manage to play two games; at other times, you might finish a whole chapter in one session. A lot of children like repeating the same stories. Once you've reached the final page, you're free to randomly select any exercise.

TIME FOR ACROBATICS

Having a full schedule is often a problem when it comes to finding time to play with your child. In this case, set times are an ideal solution. Maybe the living room is free on Wednesdays, when older brother goes to football and younger sister to drawing classes? Or maybe Grandma comes by every Saturday for an hour? Results are best when your child has your full attention during the game and distractions by others are kept to a minimum. You can, of course, involve the rest of the family by letting siblings join in with the exercise or by showing them a trick at an appropriate moment.

WELL DONE!

The importance of children receiving praise and encouragement is luckily no longer a strange concept. Try to give your child feedback on what he's doing and how he's doing it, rather than focussing on the child himself. A child who is told why he has done something well will learn much quicker. Compliments such as 'You used a lot of muscles in this exercise', or 'You landed neatly on both feet – well done', are much better encouragements than 'You're so clever'. Compliments relating to effort and approach will teach your child perseverance and help him learn from his success. Before you know it, he'll have a greater understanding of his body as well as increased motor skills, which, in turn, will promote more self-confidence. After all, when you feel at home in your body, you can take on the whole world.

And now... it's Jack's turn.

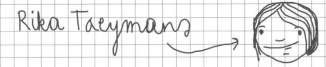

Rika Taeymans

WHO IS JACK?

Jack is five years old. He lives in a small red house with his brother, sister, mum and dad. Their house is next to a pine forest. Jack collects matchboxes and he has a grey rabbit. He loves cherries and holidays. But most of all, he adores Christmas – a time when Dad roasts the turkey and Mum lights candles. This year, the entire family is coming to dinner. Jack's brother wants to show off his football skills under the Christmas tree. His sister is going to sing a song. And as a surprise, Jack wants to perform an acrobatics routine. He has been practising really hard. Luckily, he has more than enough training partners: Mum, Dad, Jack's brother and Rabbit all want to take part in the pyramid.

Will you practise too?

Who are your training partners?

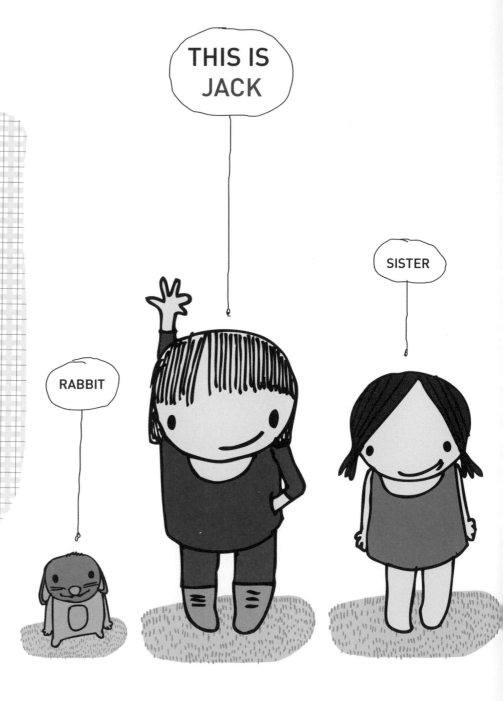

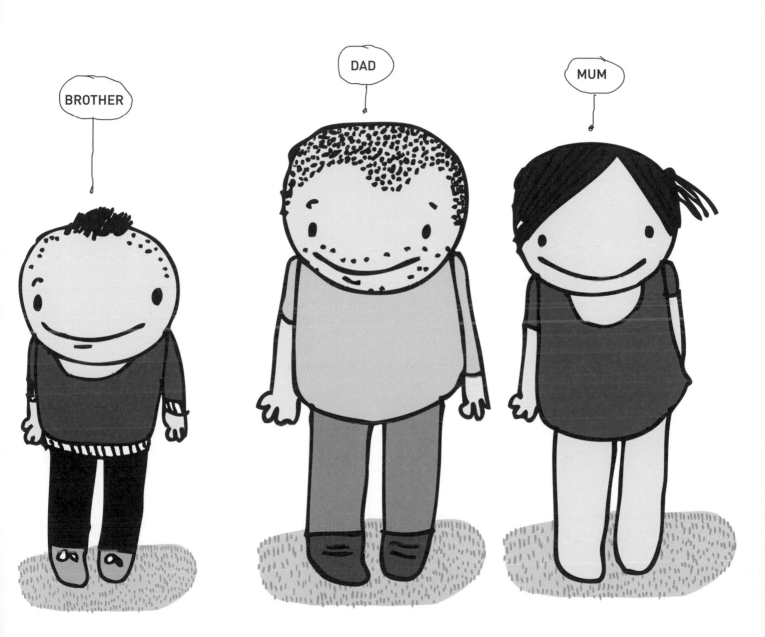

READY TO
START?

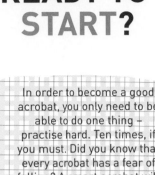

In order to become a good acrobat, you only need to be able to do one thing – practise hard. Ten times, if you must. Did you know that every acrobat has a fear of falling? A smart acrobat will only climb a pyramid when he is absolutely sure he's ready to try. Jack and Dad practise their games every weekend. Most of the time, they only play one game, but sometimes they do as many as four. This way, they strengthen their muscles and learn to be careful. Once they master these games, they're ready for the real acrobatics.

Want to know more about the theory behind these games? See page 68

Want to know more about the theory behind these games? See page 68

KEY TO SYMBOLS USED IN THE EXERCISES

   Against: these exercises focus on strength, concentration and self-confidence

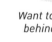   **With:** these games focus on trust, responsibility and relaxation

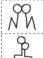   **Togeher:** cooperation is the main focus here

   Board: they learn to tighten their upper bodies

   Ball: they learn to tuck themselves into a tight ball around their core

   Free flow: they learn to relax their upper bodies

   Role changing: where possible, roles are reversed

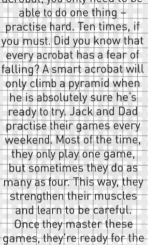

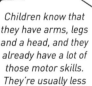

During training, you'll learn much more than you think. Each game has symbols denoting the purpose of the exercise.

Children know that they have arms, legs and a head, and they already have a lot of those motor skills. They're usually less aware of their upper bodies.

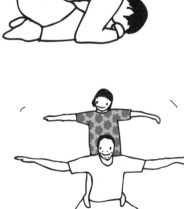

soft grass

soft carpet

PREPARING THE PISTE

You can practise acrobatics virtually anywhere. Where are the softest places in your house? The carpet? The grass? Is that old mattress still in the attic? Or maybe that duvet is perfect to put on the wooden floor?

Jack collects all the pillows in the house to build a soft practice piste. Mum wants a pillow to put under her head – and Dad, for under his bottom. Socks can make you slip and slide all over the place, so it's best to take them off. Mum rolls them up into a neat little ball. Dad checks to see whether there's anything on which he can bump his head. Jack makes sure that Rabbit isn't in the way. Now all that's left to do is to move the coffee table out of the way and the piste is ready!

soft mattress

soft duvet

socks off!

move the coffee table out of the way

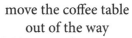

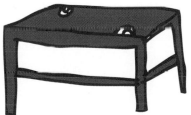

pillows to construct a practice piste

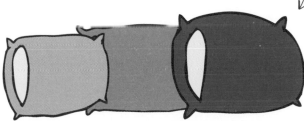

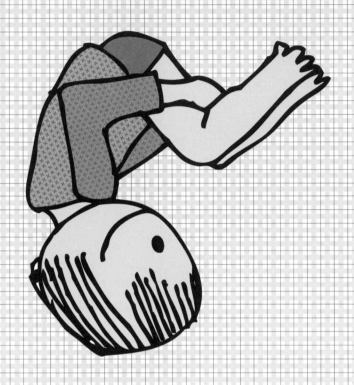

SOMERSAULTS

Somersaults are super fun. They toss you from under to over and from side to side. Can you tuck yourself into a tight little ball, like a curled-up hedgehog? Like a tiny bit of scrunched up paper? Then you're ready to spin through the air like a tennis ball. A somersault isn't always successful at first try. But once you've practised a few times, it's as easy as putting on your socks.

THE HORSE HAS AN ITCH

Sometimes Dad arrives home early from work. Then Jack gets to ride on his back. With a pat on the shoulder, Jack steers his horse around the room. Left! Right! Under the table!

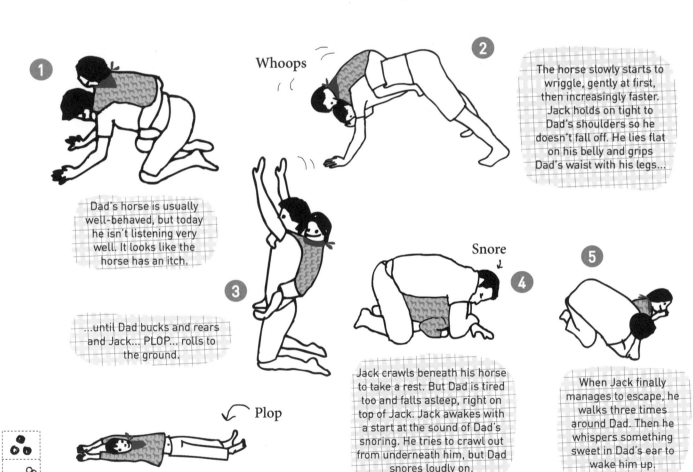

1

Dad's horse is usually well-behaved, but today he isn't listening very well. It looks like the horse has an itch.

Whoops

2

The horse slowly starts to wriggle, gently at first, then increasingly faster. Jack holds on tight to Dad's shoulders so he doesn't fall off. He lies flat on his belly and grips Dad's waist with his legs...

3

...until Dad bucks and rears and Jack... PLOP... rolls to the ground.

Plop

Snore

4

Jack crawls beneath his horse to take a rest. But Dad is tired too and falls asleep, right on top of Jack. Jack awakes with a start at the sound of Dad's snoring. He tries to crawl out from underneath him, but Dad snores loudly on.

5

When Jack finally manages to escape, he walks three times around Dad. Then he whispers something sweet in Dad's ear to wake him up.

What do you whisper into your dad's ear to wake him up?

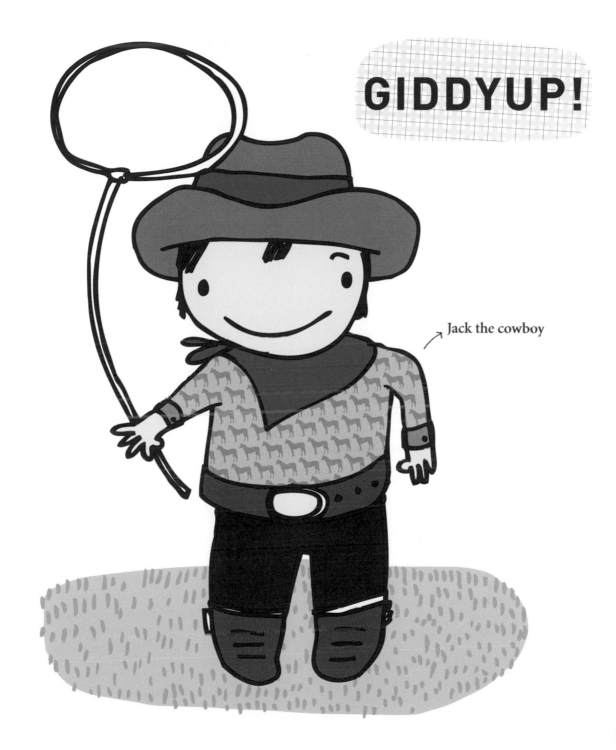

GIDDYUP!

Jack the cowboy

ROLLING SNOWBALLS

Jack loves the snow. He likes the feeling of snowflakes melting on his tongue. And he has thrown at least a hundred snowballs already – lots and lots at his brother and one at Rabbit as well. Ha ha! When the snow has melted, Jack pretends to be a snowball himself.

1 He kneels and makes himself as small as possible. 'Mum, will you roll me through the snow?'

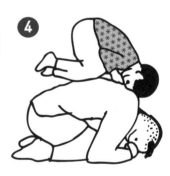

2 Mum rolls Jack across the floor. He stays in a tight ball, his nose glued to his knees. When he rolls onto his back, Jack tries his best not to let his snowball fall apart. Mum rolls him all around the room until she grows tired.

Then Mum gets to pretend to be a snowball. This is the largest snowball Jack has ever seen. He rolls Mum across the floor and feels his arm muscles grow.

3

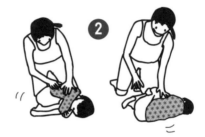

'Shall we make a snowman?' Mum rolls Jack's brother into a large snowball. Then, it's Jack's turn. Could Mum please put him on top of his brother?

4

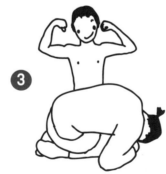

5 The snowman remains standing until the sun comes out. Then Jack and his brother start to melt until they're flat on the ground, on top of each other.

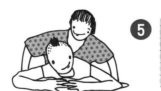

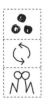

✳ Could you build a snowman with three balls? Who gets to go on top? Dad? Or Rabbit?

CRACK!

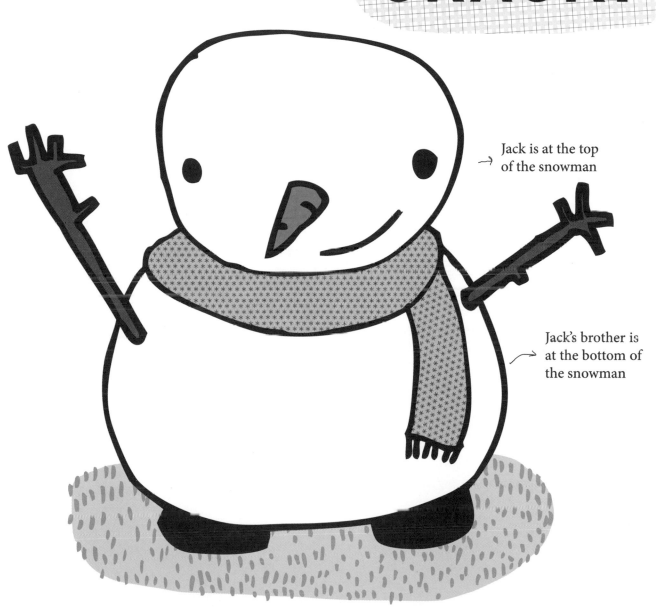

Jack is at the top of the snowman

Jack's brother is at the bottom of the snowman

TUMBLING OUT OF THE WHEELBARROW

There are two tall apple trees in Jack's garden. In spring, a thousand white flowers bloom in them. And in the autumn, hundreds of apples fall onto the grass. Jack and his sister help to collect the apples, so that Mum can make applesauce from them. Mmm...

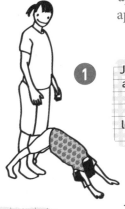

1 Jack pretends to be a wheelbarrow. He puts his hands on the ground and looks past his belly to his feet.

2 Mum stands in between his legs and grabs the top of his legs, just above his knees.

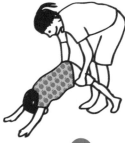

3 While she lifts his legs, Jack uses his arms to support his body firmly. He keeps his belly raised. Then, Mum can start to drive him around. Jack moves forward on his hands.

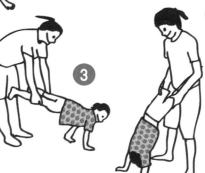

4 As soon as the wheelbarrow is full, Mum lifts Jack's legs higher – almost into a handstand.

5 Jack looks at his belly, tucks his head in and rolls from the wheelbarrow like a round apple.

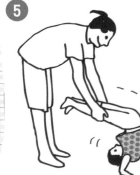

✳ Does your wheelbarrow move backward as well?

VROOM!

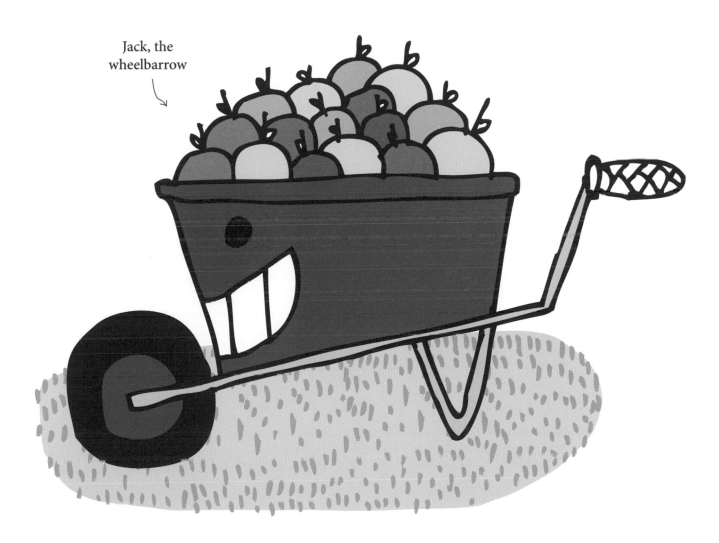

Jack, the wheelbarrow

THE VERY CLEVER PRESENT

Tomorrow is Jack's grandmother's birthday. She loves gifts.
As a surprise, Jack wraps himself up as a really pretty present.

1 His arms and legs are four big bows that keep the package tightly closed. But Grandma is very curious. When nobody is looking, she tries to sneak a peek at her wrapped present. Jack feels her fingers scratch softly at the paper. She tugs increasingly harder on the bows.

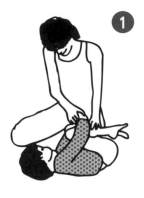

2 'No! Your birthday isn't until tomorrow. I won't open yet!' Grandma carefully lifts the present, to feel how heavy it is. Can she hear what's inside? But Jack is clever and strong, and he keeps the four bows tightly closed.

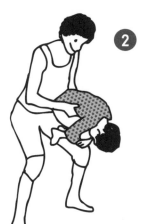

3 The following day, Grandma gets to open her present. The bows are no longer tight and open with ease. The present flops open when all the ribbons are flat on the ground. Jack now looks like a big, beautiful star. 'Happy birthday, Grandma!'

4 Jack wishes it was his birthday too. 'Grandma, would you wrap yourself up for me? I would like to open a present, too!'

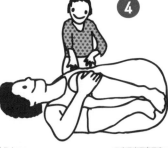
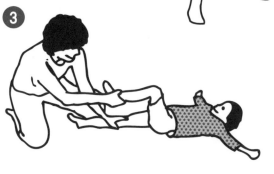

What's in your present? Can you show us?

CRUMPLE!

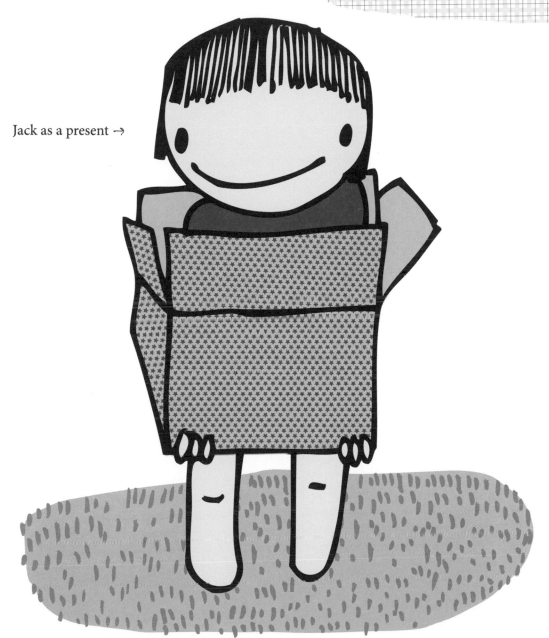

Jack as a present →

THE WHAT'S UP SOMERSAULT

Sometimes, Jack's sister and Dad cuddle so hard that they almost become tangled in a knot. And his Mum and brother give each other so many kisses that Jack has lost count. Jack's favourite greeting is 'What's up?' 'Hey Dad, What's up?' 'Hey Jack, everything's OK!'

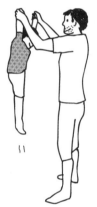

1 Dad holds up two thumbs. Jack grabs hold of them and Dad's big hands close around Jack's small hands. If Dad's thumbs are strong enough, Jack can hang on to them while his legs dangle in the air.

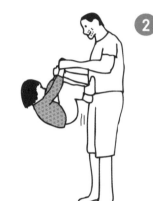

2 Using his feet, Jack walks up Dad's body. One step at a time, via his knees and over his stomach.

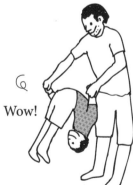

Wow!

3 When he's all the way at the top, Jack tucks himself into a small ball and tumbles backwards into a somersault. Whee!

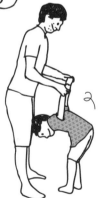

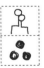

Have you got the hang of this? Then try to do the somersault from Dad's thumbs. First, jump really high with your legs in the air, until you almost touch the ceiling. If you can do that, tuck yourself into a little ball at the highest point. You will automatically tumble backwards and land on your feet. Can you do this without touching Dad's stomach?

WHEE!

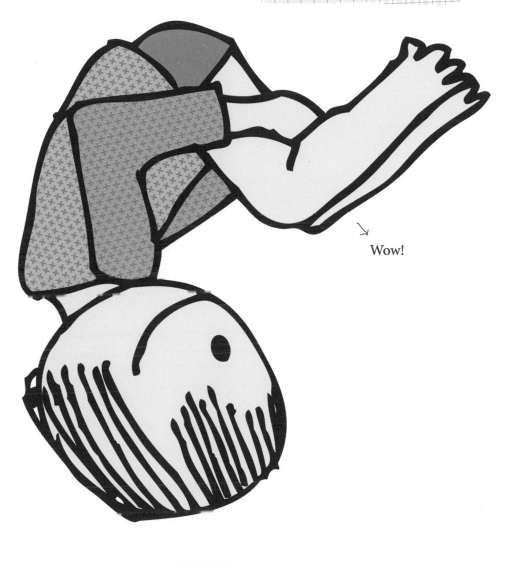

Wow!

THE NOSE-TICKLE SOMERSAULT

Jack can see the whole world from Mum's shoulders. He sees Rabbit nibbling on some grass in the neighbours' garden. He sees dust on the kitchen lamp. And isn't that France, all the way in the distance? Or wait, is it China perhaps? For Jack to land on his feet, he and Mum have thought up a real acrobatic somersault. Watch!

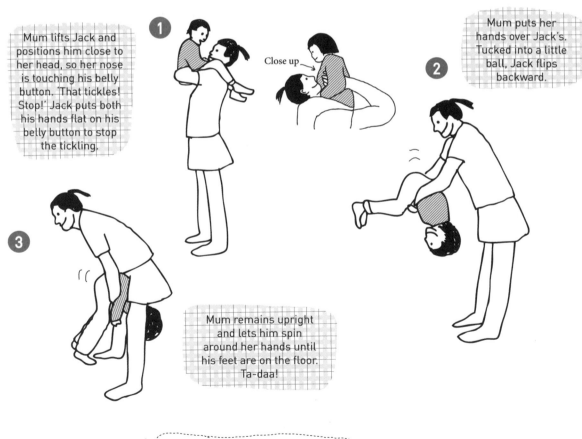

1 Mum lifts Jack and positions him close to her head, so her nose is touching his belly button. 'That tickles! Stop!' Jack puts both his hands flat on his belly button to stop the tickling.

Close up

2 Mum puts her hands over Jack's. Tucked into a little ball, Jack flips backward.

3 Mum remains upright and lets him spin around her hands until his feet are on the floor. Ta-daa!

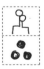

What can you see from Mum's shoulders?

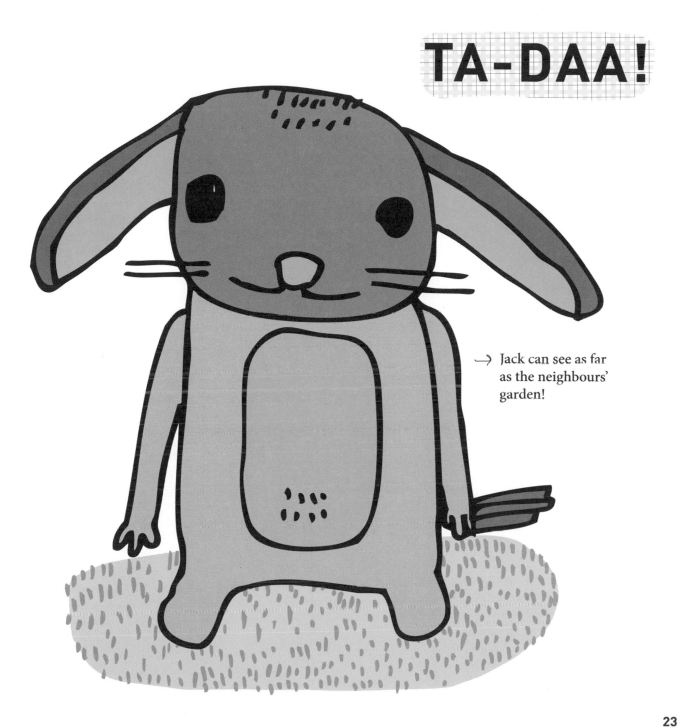

TA-DAA!

→ Jack can see as far as the neighbours' garden!

23

THE WALL SOMERSAULT

Mum draws a line on the kitchen wall, just above Jack's head. This way, Jack can see how much he has grown – and how small he was just last year. 'Ha ha, so small!' His sister's lines are lower and his brother's lines are way up high. Jack hopes that one day he'll reach the ceiling. But being small is fine, too, because small acrobats can somersault over their own heads. It's true.

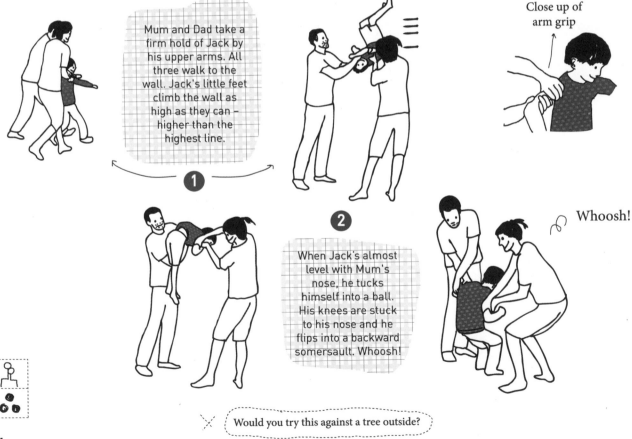

Mum and Dad take a firm hold of Jack by his upper arms. All three walk to the wall. Jack's little feet climb the wall as high as they can – higher than the highest line.

1

Close up of arm grip

2

When Jack's almost level with Mum's nose, he tucks himself into a ball. His knees are stuck to his nose and he flips into a backward somersault. Whoosh!

Whoosh!

Would you try this against a tree outside?

TA-DAA!

— BROTHER

— JACK

→ Jack has grown!

— SISTER

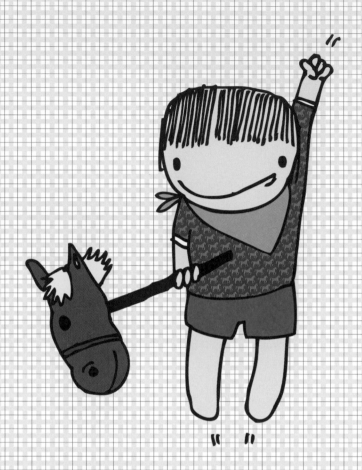

PYRAMIDS

Pyramids are very difficult to do. Who will be at the top? And who will support everyone else at the base? It takes some measuring and figuring out for each acrobat to find their place. After some wobbly moments, they all stay strong. Only then does the pyramid hold firm. Can you make yourself as strong as a brick in a castle wall? Or as stiff as a card in a house of cards? Then we can start to build. Do you think we can reach the ceiling?

THE SLEEPING COW

Jack's dad tells a lot of stories. Once, when they were at the seaside, he told Jack he swam all the way to France. And sometimes he says that beer makes the hairs on his chest shine. He also says that cows sleep standing up, and that you can tip them over very easily. Jack isn't sure if he should believe that one. Dad is on his hands and knees and pretends to be a cow that has fallen asleep. He dreams of green meadows full of little calves.

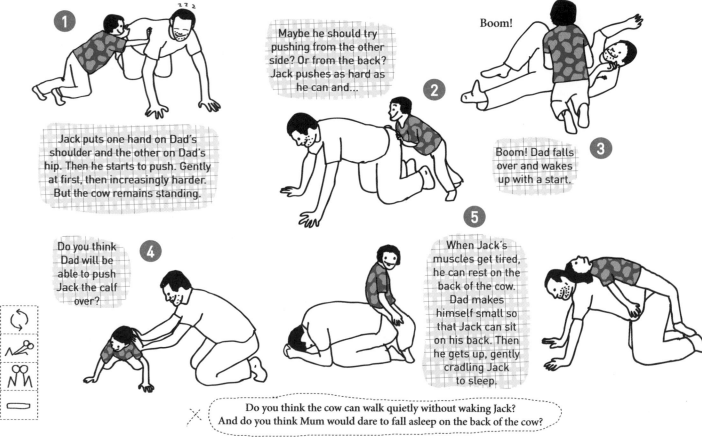

1 Jack puts one hand on Dad's shoulder and the other on Dad's hip. Then he starts to push. Gently at first, then increasingly harder. But the cow remains standing.

Maybe he should try pushing from the other side? Or from the back? Jack pushes as hard as he can and...

2

Boom!

3 Boom! Dad falls over and wakes up with a start.

Do you think Dad will be able to push Jack the calf over?

4

5 When Jack's muscles get tired, he can rest on the back of the cow. Dad makes himself small so that Jack can sit on his back. Then he gets up, gently cradling Jack to sleep.

Do you think the cow can walk quietly without waking Jack? And do you think Mum would dare to fall asleep on the back of the cow?

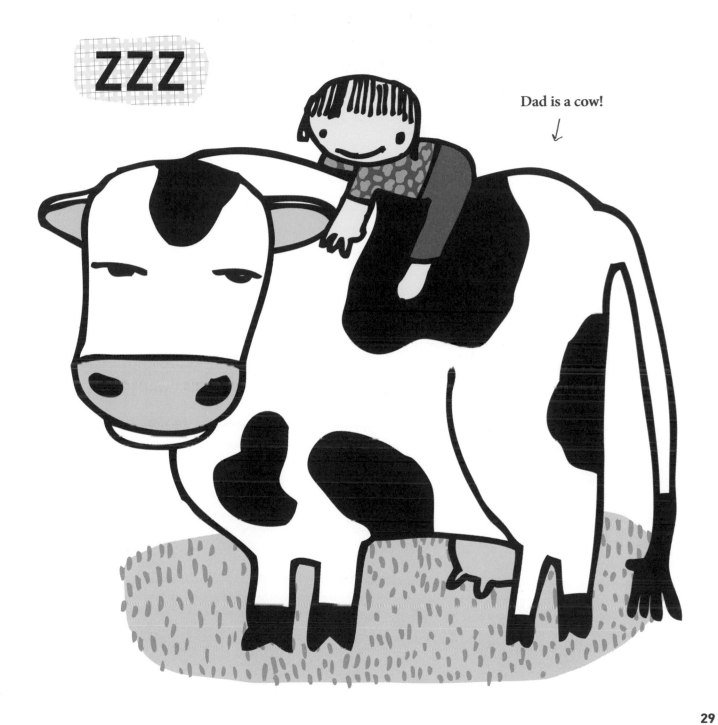

ZZZ

Dad is a cow!

AUNTIE'S TIGER RUG

There's a large, striped tiger rug in Auntie's hallway. She vacuums it daily. She even cleans underneath it once a year. And sometimes she finds little treasures: a lost ring... a match... a bit of fluff that looks like a ghost... But the carpet is so heavy that Auntie can't lift it by herself. Luckily, Jack has big, strong muscles. 'I'll help!'

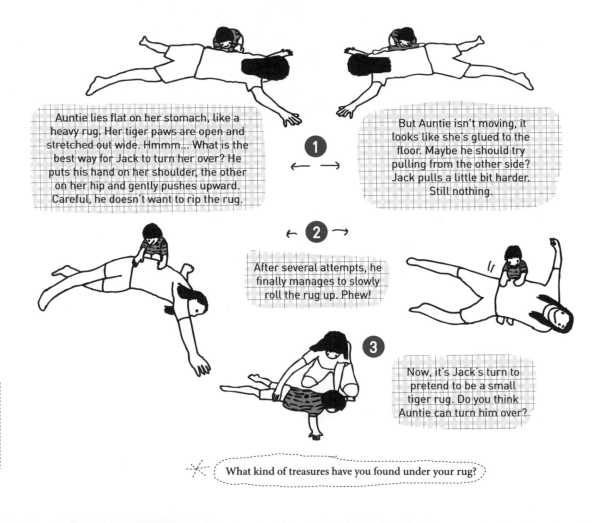

1

Auntie lies flat on her stomach, like a heavy rug. Her tiger paws are open and stretched out wide. Hmmm... What is the best way for Jack to turn her over? He puts his hand on her shoulder, the other on her hip and gently pushes upward. Careful, he doesn't want to rip the rug.

But Auntie isn't moving, it looks like she's glued to the floor. Maybe he should try pulling from the other side? Jack pulls a little bit harder. Still nothing.

2

After several attempts, he finally manages to slowly roll the rug up. Phew!

3

Now, it's Jack's turn to pretend to be a small tiger rug. Do you think Auntie can turn him over?

What kind of treasures have you found under your rug?

30

Jack, the rug

ROAR!

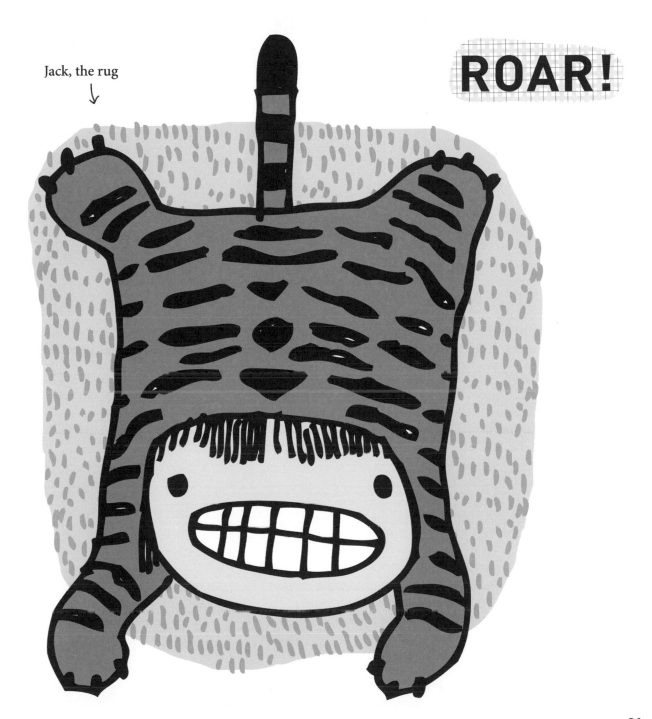

THE STRONG ROCK

Every summer, Jack goes to the seaside for a week. His sister collects shells. And his brother waits until Dad falls asleep so he can bury him under a heap of sand. Jack likes counting waves. Mum won't let him go out too far in the deep water. 'Nothing is stronger than the sea!' she says. 'But what about rocks?' Jack asks.

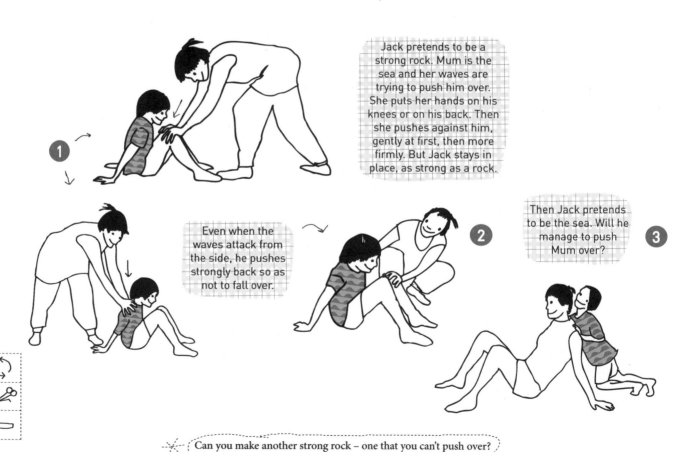

1 Jack pretends to be a strong rock. Mum is the sea and her waves are trying to push him over. She puts her hands on his knees or on his back. Then she pushes against him, gently at first, then more firmly. But Jack stays in place, as strong as a rock.

Even when the waves attack from the side, he pushes strongly back so as not to fall over.

2

3 Then Jack pretends to be the sea. Will he manage to push Mum over?

Can you make another strong rock – one that you can't push over?

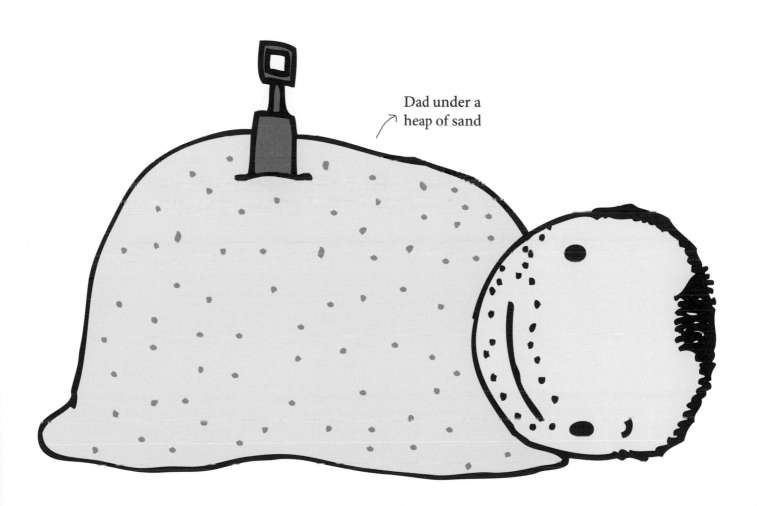

SWISH! SWISH!

Dad under a
heap of sand

THE BLOWN-DOWN TREE TRUNK

Last night, a heavy storm raged over Jack's house. He crawled into his brother's bed and together they counted the claps of thunder. In the woods behind the house, blown-down tree trunks are scattered like bundles of Mikado sticks. The forester is sad. 'We'll help you replant the trees!' Jack and his brother say.

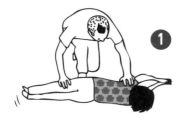

1 Jack lies on the ground and pretends to be a tall pine tree. His brother rolls him to an open clearing in the forest.

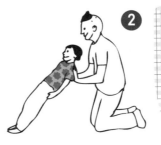

2 His brother tries to push Jack upright. Jack remains as stiff as a board until he is upright. Jack can feel how his brother is replanting his roots with scoops of earth.

Dad checks if Jack's tree is sturdy and gently pulls on his shoulders. Oh dear, Jack falls backwards, stiff as a board, right into Dad's hands. But Jack also falls forward, to the left and to the right. Dad catches him each and every time. Jack's brother digs a deeper hole. He continues until Jack stands as solid as the Eiffel Tower. Now he can withstand any gust of wind. Try and blow him down!

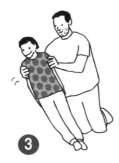

3

Jack crawls into the highest tree in the forest to see where the other fallen trees are. Dad pretends to be the tree, his feet set wide apart and his knees bent. Jack puts his feet in Dad's groin and climbs up high until he is upright against the tree trunk. 'Ah ha, there are some pine trees lying around in the distance!'

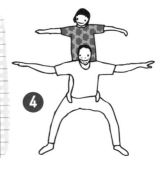

4

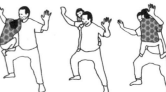

Can you climb all the way up the tree trunk without touching the ground? Or under the roots of the tree?

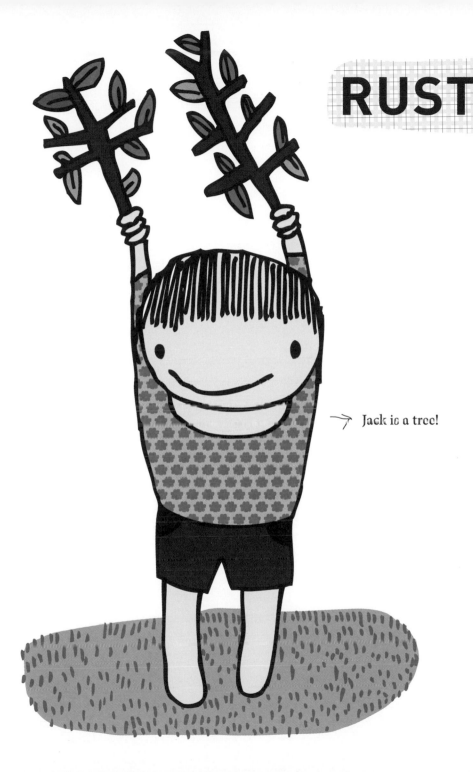

RUSTLE!

→ Jack is a tree!

THE PONY PYRAMID

There's a brown pony in the neighbours' garden. He likes to eat grass and uses his tail to swat the flies from his back. When Jack turns six, the neighbours will let him ride the pony. In the meantime, Jack practises with Dad. They circle the whole kitchen. Jack can even stand upright on Dad's back.

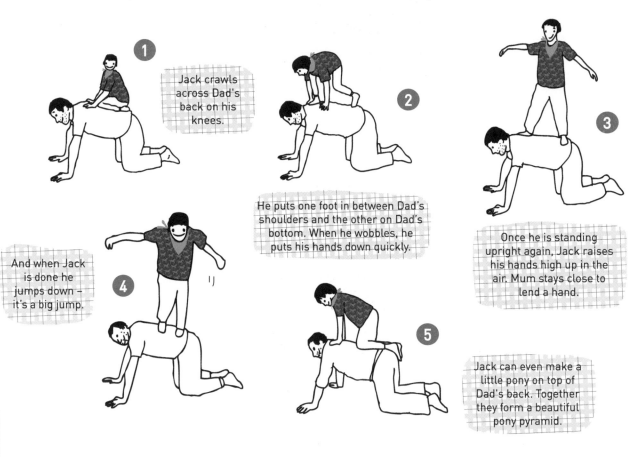

1 Jack crawls across Dad's back on his knees.

2 He puts one foot in between Dad's shoulders and the other on Dad's bottom. When he wobbles, he puts his hands down quickly.

3 Once he is standing upright again, Jack raises his hands high up in the air. Mum stays close to lend a hand.

4 And when Jack is done he jumps down – it's a big jump.

5 Jack can even make a little pony on top of Dad's back. Together they form a beautiful pony pyramid.

Can you think of another way to get down?

36

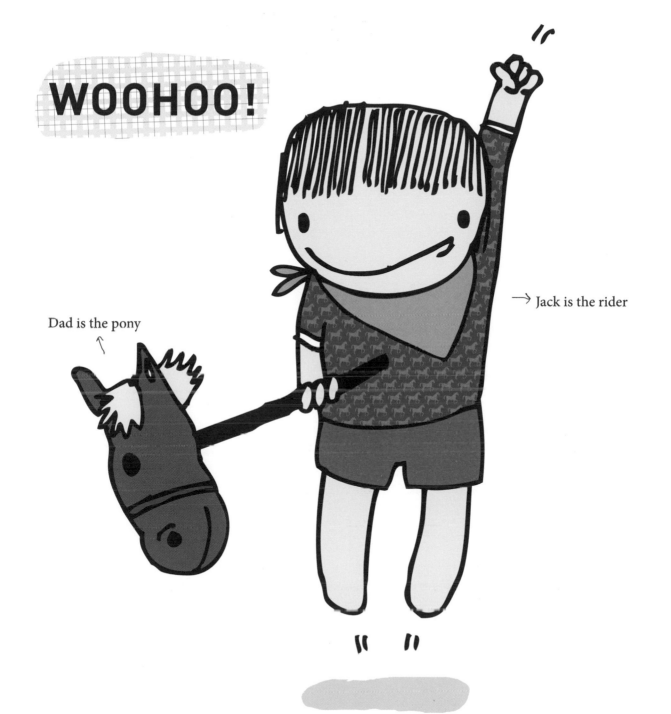

THE FLAG

Jack loves looking at flags. They flutter as if they want to fly away in the wind. His favourite flag is the Vietnamese flag, which has a large star in the middle of it. If he were a flag, he would be a European flag, a blue one with yellow stars; or a white one with pink dots, above his sister's doll house.

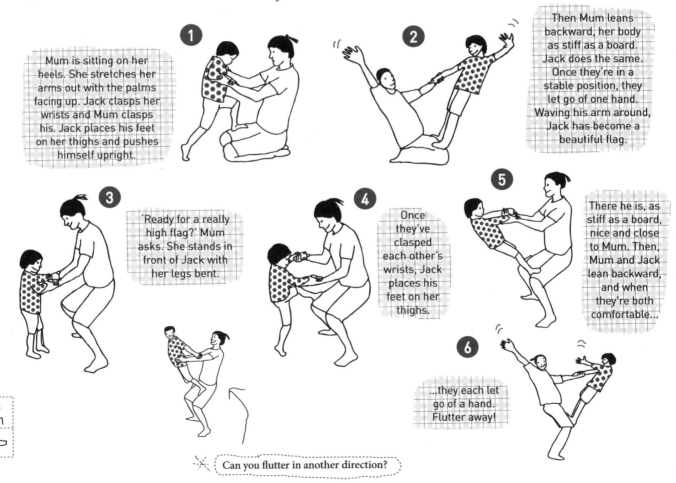

1 Mum is sitting on her heels. She stretches her arms out with the palms facing up. Jack clasps her wrists and Mum clasps his. Jack places his feet on her thighs and pushes himself upright.

2 Then Mum leans backward, her body as stiff as a board. Jack does the same. Once they're in a stable position, they let go of one hand. Waving his arm around, Jack has become a beautiful flag.

3 'Ready for a really high flag?' Mum asks. She stands in front of Jack with her legs bent.

4 Once they've clasped each other's wrists, Jack places his feet on her thighs.

5 There he is, as stiff as a board, nice and close to Mum. Then, Mum and Jack lean backward, and when they're both comfortable...

6 ...they each let go of a hand. Flutter away!

Can you flutter in another direction?

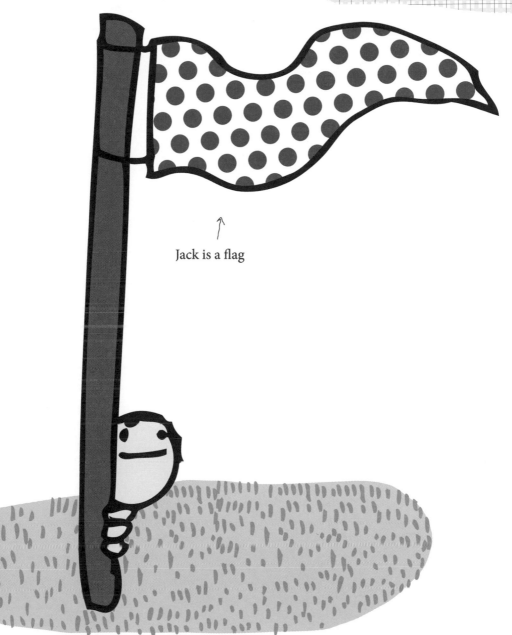

THE BUNK BED

Jack sleeps in a room with his brother. His brother's bed is near the window and Jack's bed is near the door. Jack has asked Santa Claus for a bunk bed. Then, he can sleep on top. Maybe it'll help if they build a bunk bed themselves?

1

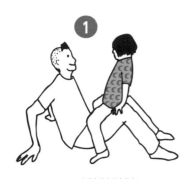

Jack's brother is the taller. He sits on his bottom. Jack sits on his brother's knees so they're facing each other. Then he puts his feet on his brother's shoulders.

2

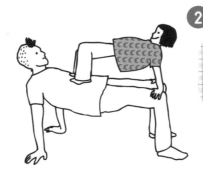

'One, two, three!' his brother whispers, and they both push their bellies upward.

Then they build another bunk bed, this time with their heads facing the same direction. Will they succeed?

3

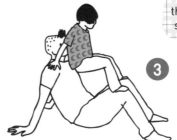

4 Dad wants to be in the bunk bed as well. He has the lower bed. Mum helps Jack and his brother. Do you think three bunks will work?

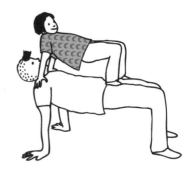

 Can a bunk bed remain upright on three legs?

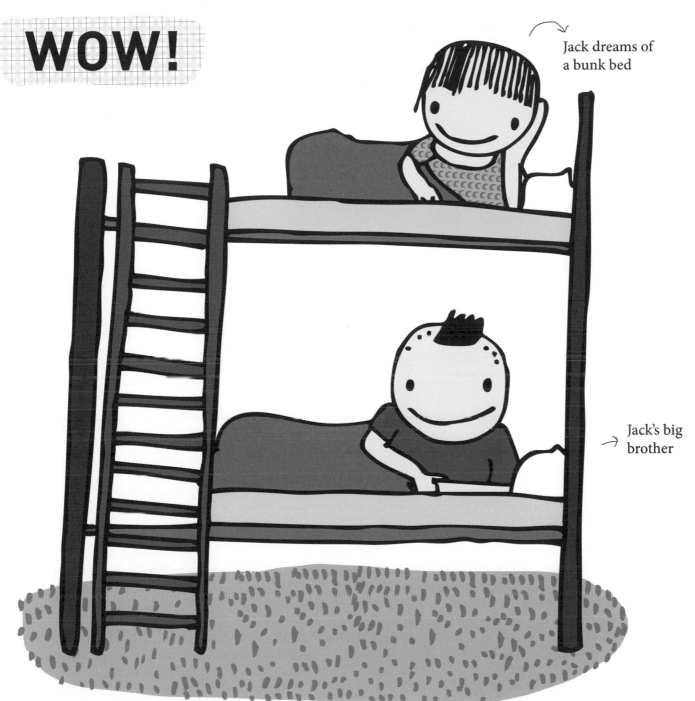

WOW!

Jack dreams of a bunk bed

Jack's big brother

THE BEST LADDER

Jack wishes he was as tall as his brother, who can already reach the biscuits in the top kitchen cabinet if he stands on a chair. Jack is only as tall as Mum's belly button. Luckily, Dad likes helping Jack. Jack gets to climb up his dad until he is taller than everyone else and can easily reach the biscuit tin!

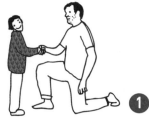

1

Dad kneels on his left knee with his right foot planted firmly on the floor in front of him and his leg bent at a right angle. 'Ready?' he asks. 'Ready!' Jack replies. They shake hands and keep a firm grip.

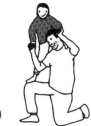

2

But no doubt it's going to be a sweaty business. They use their left hand to wipe the sweat from their brow.

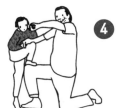

3

Then they hook their left hands together, keeping the thumbs down.

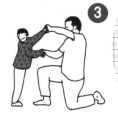

4

Jack climbs up as if he is climbing a ladder. The first rung is the easiest.

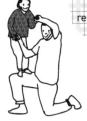

5

Jack climbs onto Dad's thigh, placing both feet behind Dad's knee.

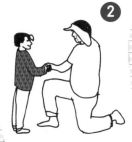

6

The next rung of the ladder is a bit more difficult – Jack puts his left foot on Dad's left shoulder.

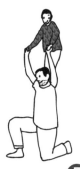

7

Dad pulls Jack up with both arms. Jack places his other foot on Dad's right shoulder and stands upright, with his feet close to Dad's neck. He has never been this tall.

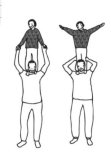

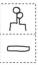

 Have you practised a lot? Then you can try to raise your hands in the air while Dad holds you by the backs of your knees and presses your legs against his head.

UP! UP! UP!

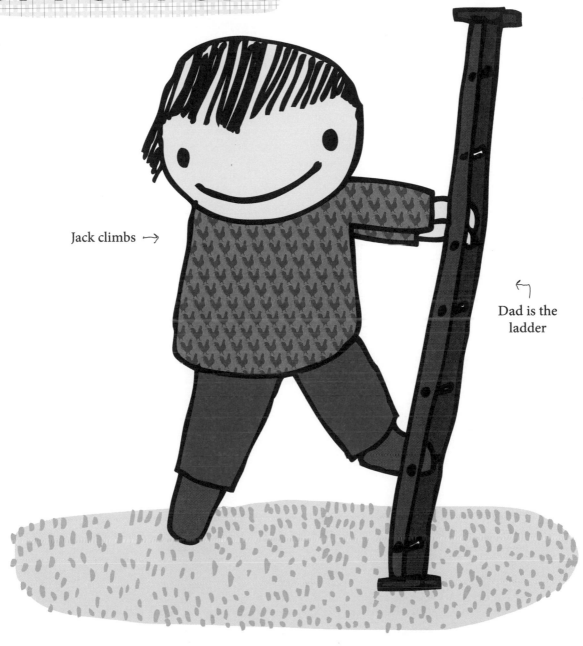

Jack climbs →

← Dad is the ladder

THE BUCKING DONKEY

Jack's sister loves donkeys. Sometimes Dad lifts her up so she can stroke their nose. But you should never stand behind a donkey. That's what Dad says. You see, when donkeys are angry, they kick their hind legs backward really hard.

1 Jack and his sister play at being angry donkeys. They are on their hands and knees bucking with their hind legs. Bucking is fun!

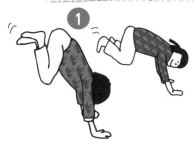

2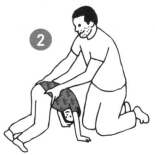

Jack kicks his legs so high that he's almost in a handstand. Maybe he'll succeed with Dad's help. Dad stands in front of Jack and takes hold of Jack's hips.

3 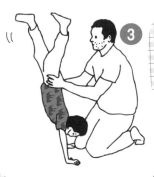 Jack bucks as high as he can and Dad helps him into a handstand.

4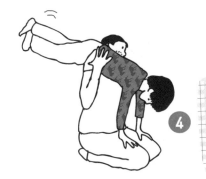

Ready for a handstand pyramid? Dad sits on his heels. Jack stands behind Dad and raises his arms in the air. Jack stands as stiff as a board and Dad lifts him over his shoulder until Jack's hands rest on his thighs.

5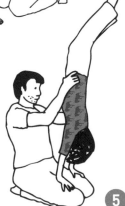

Jack remains nice and stiff and Dad helps him into a handstand. Brilliant!

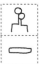

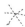 Within five seconds, Jack's face is as red as a beetroot. How long can you stay in a handstand before your face turns red?

HEE HAW

Jack is a
bucking donkey
↑

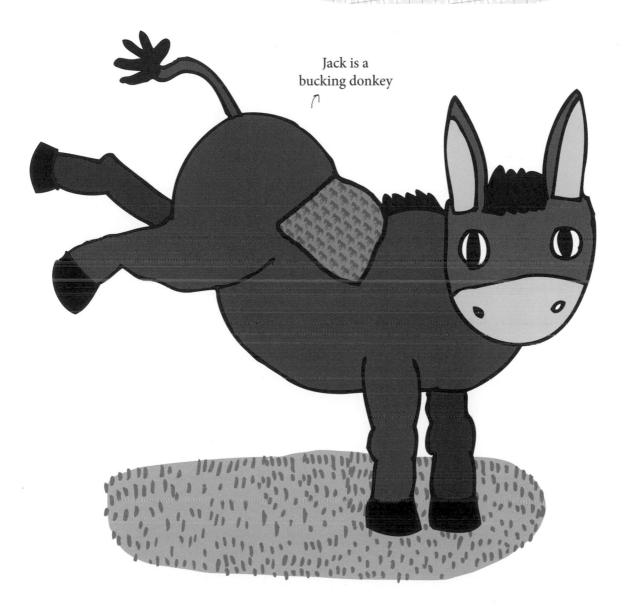

THE LOOKOUT

Jack has his brother's old bike – a beautiful red one with a big bell. He learnt to ride it last summer. He loves to cycle to his Grandma's house. It's his favourite route. He has to cross two bridges, cycle past at least twenty cows and cross one big hill to get there. There's a fine lookout on the top of the hill, where Jack can rest and have a glass of juice.

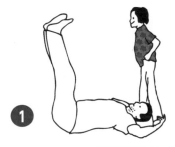

1

When it rains, Jack and Dad cycle at home on the mat. Dad lies on his back, his hands next to his ears. Then he raises his legs so Jack can grab his feet. Jack carefully places his feet in Dad's hands. Dad holds Jack's feet by the heels.

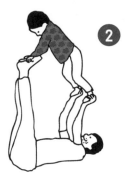

2

'One, two three!' counts Dad. Jack jumps up in the air. At the same time, Dad raises and stretches his arms and... whoosh! Jack is standing on Dad's outstretched arms with straight legs. 'Ready to cycle, Jack?' Dad asks. Jack slowly starts to pedal, making small circular movements with Dad's hands. Cycling uphill is going to be even more difficult, but Jack is strong.

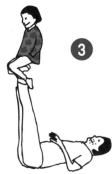

3

When they reach the top of the hill, Dad places his feet at the back of Jack's knees. Jack sits upright, his bottom securely supported by Dad's feet. A fine lookout!

4

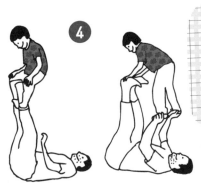

To climb down, Jack grabs Dad's feet and Dad grabs Jack's heels. Jack frees his legs and places his feet again in Dad's hands. Dad gently lowers Jack to the floor.

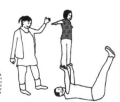

When you've practised this for a while, try standing upright in your dad's hand like a tall lookout tower after you've cycled. It's best if your mum stands behind you. Are you ready to try without using your hands?

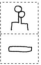

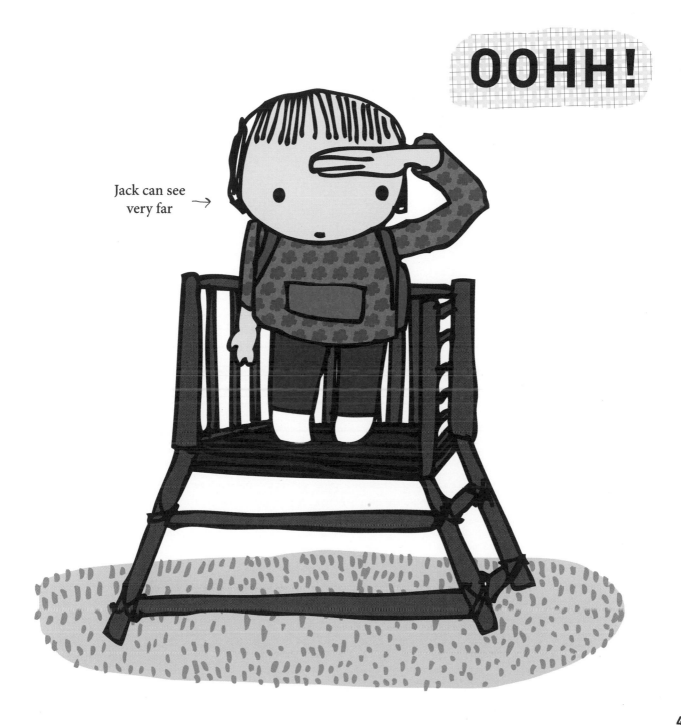

Jack can see very far →

OOHH!

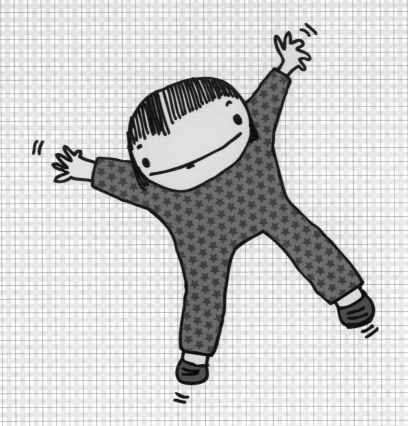

FREE FLOW

Nothing is more delightful than flowing freely through the air: drifting briefly through the clouds or gently swaying from side to side; relaxed and loose like your underwear in the washing machine; like an autumn leaf in wild winds. You don't need any skills for this. But sometimes, doing nothing is harder than you think.

IN THE
ROCKING CHAIR

Jack's Dad has a large wooden rocking chair. He rocks in it for hours,
backward and forward. Sometimes Jack gets to rock back and forth, too.

1 Jack crawls onto Dad's lap and sits in between his legs. Dad grips him firmly under his knees and Jack tucks himself into a sturdy little ball.

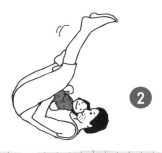

2 Then, with an arched back, Dad rolls backward. Whee! For a moment, Jack's feet dangle high up in the air. They rock backward and forward no less than ten times. 1...2...3...4...5...6...7...8...9...10!

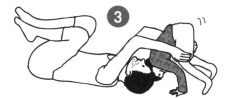

Suddenly, the rocking chair tips so far back that Jack rolls out like a ball. Dad doesn't understand – where did Jack go?

3

'Tee-hee, here I am! Wait, I'll come back!' Dad raises his arms up in the air and Jack tumbles over his shoulder, back into the rocking chair. With his free hand, Dad helps Jack tuck his head inward. With his other hand, he makes sure Jack stays tight in his neat little ball, until they're both upright and can continue rocking. When Dad gets dizzy, he takes a break and lies down flat on his back. Jack crawls onto Dad's chest. Can he hear Dad's heartbeat?

4

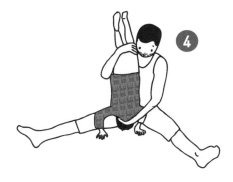

What if the rocking chair suddenly changes into a prison? Can you escape when your dad's legs and arms hold you tight? When you're free, walk three times around your dad. Then Dad gets to go in prison.

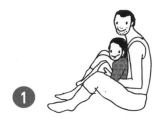

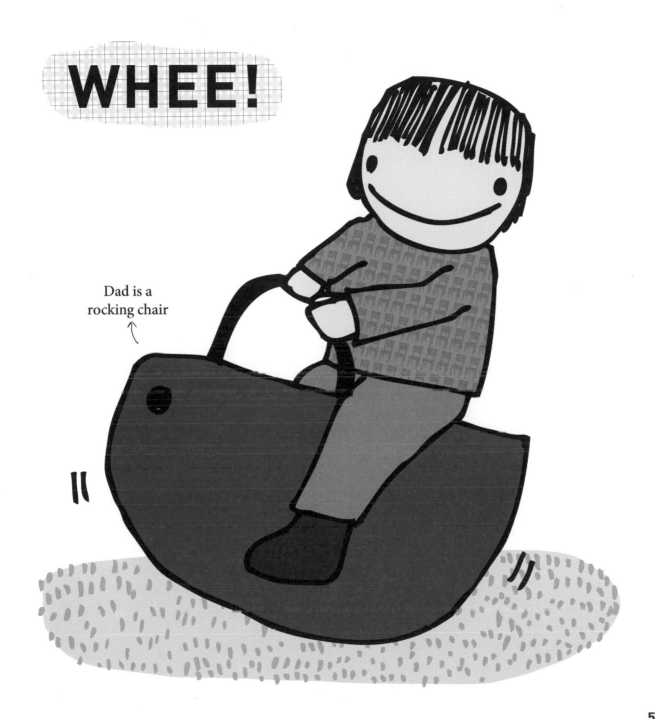

SPINNING LIKE A PLANET

Jack already knows three planets: Earth, Mars and Jupiter. Dad says the planets constantly spin around each other as well as on their own axis. Jack gets dizzy thinking about it. Dad and Jack are spinning around on their own axis as well as around each other and stagger around the room.

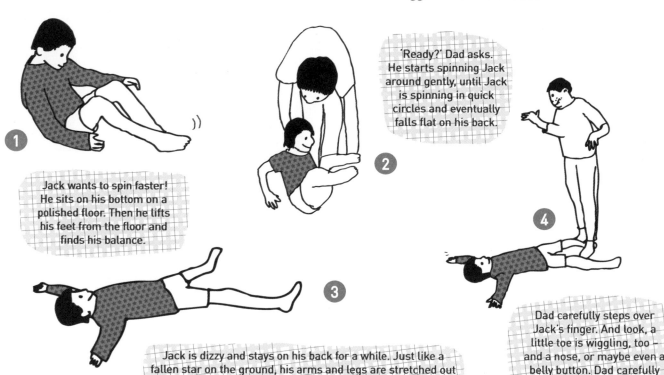

1 Jack wants to spin faster! He sits on his bottom on a polished floor. Then he lifts his feet from the floor and finds his balance.

2 'Ready?' Dad asks. He starts spinning Jack around gently, until Jack is spinning in quick circles and eventually falls flat on his back.

3 Jack is dizzy and stays on his back for a while. Just like a fallen star on the ground, his arms and legs are stretched out to the sides. Dad is worried and takes a look – is the star still alive? Then, almost unnoticably, Jack wiggles one of his little fingers. The rest of his body remains completely still.

4 Dad carefully steps over Jack's finger. And look, a little toe is wiggling, too – and a nose, or maybe even a belly button. Dad carefully looks at what's moving and steps repeatedly over the moving parts. Jack wakes up five wiggles later. Now it's Dad's turn.

 Can you spin yourself around using just your hands?

SPIN!

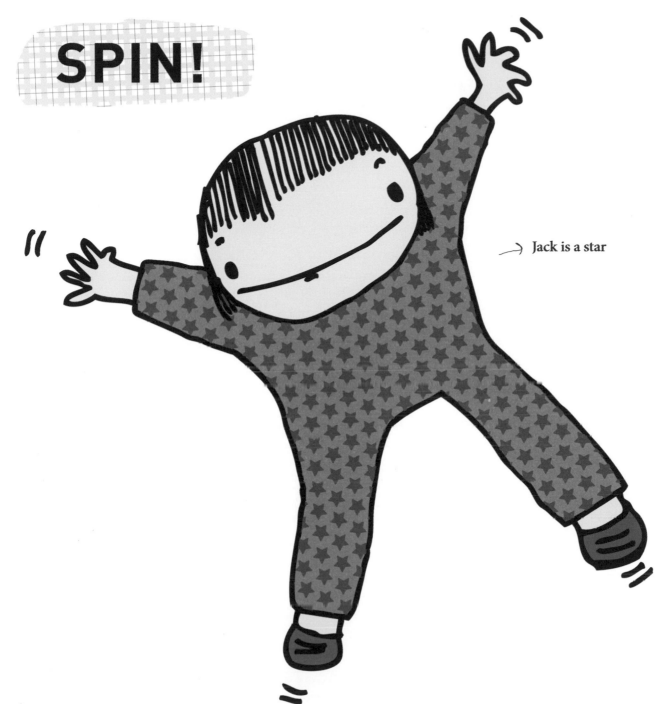

Jack is a star

THE VACUUM CLEANER

Saturday is the day for cleaning the house. Jack's brother wipes breadcrumbs off the table with a small cloth and Dad ties up the rubbish bags. Jack's sister combs Rabbit and Mum and Jack vacuum the whole house. Every bit of fluff in every corner needs to go.

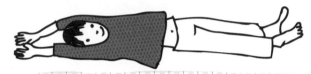

1 Jack pretends to be a vacuum cleaner, lies on his back.

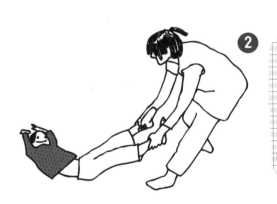

2 Mum clasps his ankles, presses the on-button and pulls the vacuum cleaner around the room. Zzzzzz! Jack is swung from side to side and sucks up everything. Every paper clip, every biscuit crumb.

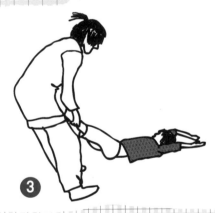

3 Sometimes the kitchen floor is so dirty that it needs a thorough clean. Mum pushes a special button that turns Jack into a floor scrubbing machine. He keeps his legs very stiff, so Mum can push him forward. Mum really works those stains, back and forth, until the floor shines like a diamond.

This only works if the floor is really smooth.
A jumper with a hood, or a blanket makes gliding around easier as well.

RRRRR!

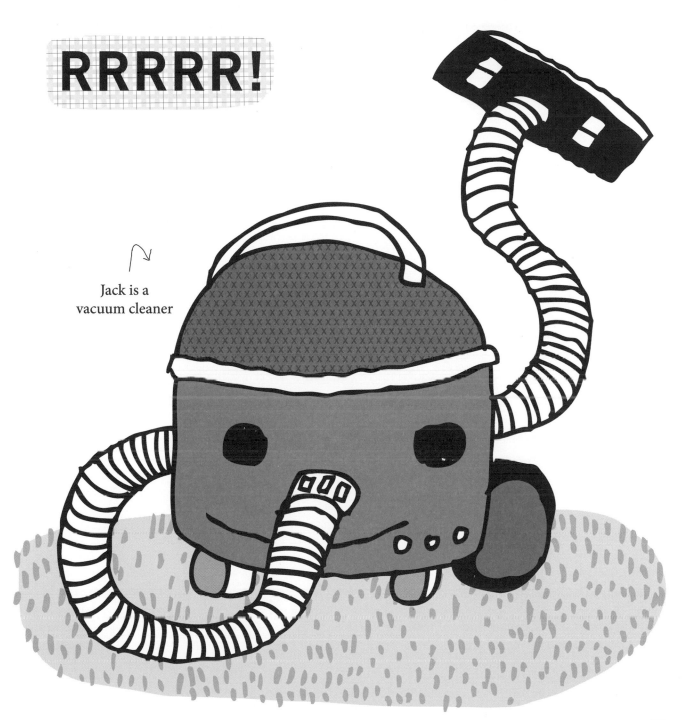

Jack is a
vacuum cleaner

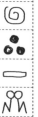

STRANDS OF SPAGHETTI

Tonight, Grandad is coming to dinner. He loves spaghetti. Jack is helping to cook and takes a packet from the cupboard. 'Is spaghetti hard or soft?' Dad asks. 'Err... hard!' 'Absolutely right,' Dad says 'But absolutely wrong at the same time. What do strands of spaghetti feel like in your mouth?' *Soft*, Jack thinks. How is that possible?

Jack is on the floor like a hard strand of spaghetti. He stretches himself out as much as he can. Dad rolls him over to the pot. Jack keeps his arms glued to his ears and his feet and legs firmly together. It's easier to roll around this way. **1**

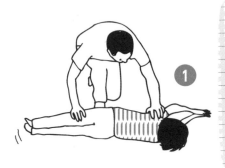

Dad lets him simmer in the pot until he is completely soft. 'Ready, Jack is done!' When Dad rolls Jack out of the pot, his arms and legs fall on the floor, completely limp. He must surely be the softest, most floppy spaghetti in the world! Rolling around is much harder now. **2**

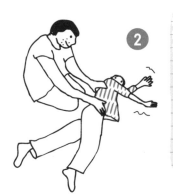

Dad prefers ravioli to spaghetti. He puts tomato sauce on Jack's stomach and folds him into a ball of ravioli. Then he turns Jack onto his knees, lifts him up and sets him down on the table. Bon appétit! Dad feasts on the Jack ravioli – it is delicious. **3**

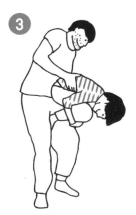

Now it's Jack's turn to munch Dad. **4**

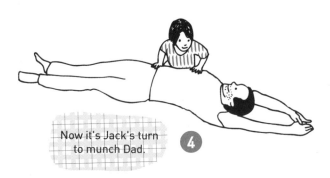

Can you create a spaghetti garland? Both of you lie on your stomach on the floor and hold each others' hands. Can you roll over together, while continuing to look at each other? For spaghetti that's already cooked and sticks to itself, lie on the floor stomach to stomach and let your dad's arms envelop you. Can you roll around the floor like this?

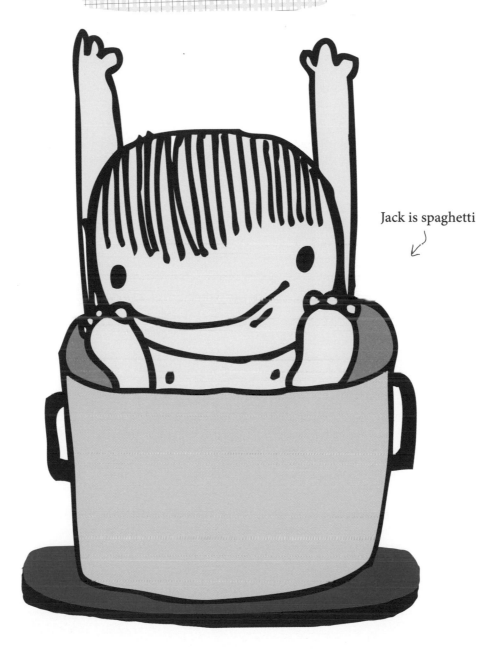

Jack is spaghetti

THE FIREMAN FREE FLOW

Jack and his sister have three babysitters. Jack likes Eva best. Her hair smells a little like apricots and she knows lots of fun games to play. When Jack gets to choose, they always pretend to be firemen.

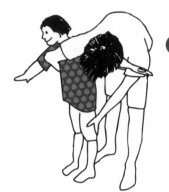

1 'Help, my room is on fire!' Jack waves his arms around frantically for help. 'Nee naw! Nee naw!' Eva rushes toward him with sirens blaring. She stands next to Jack and puts her right arm around his waist. Her left hand grips his left hip.

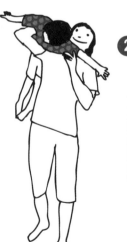

2 With a great big swoop she lifts him up and tosses him over her right shoulder. Unconscious, Jack dangles over her shoulders. 'Hey, Jack, are you still alive?'

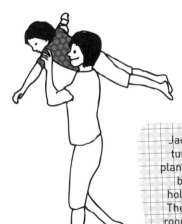

3 Jack blinks. Then he turns himself into a plane on Eva's shoulder by stretching and holding his body stiff. They twirl around the room. 'Yippee! I'm still alive. Eva saved me!'

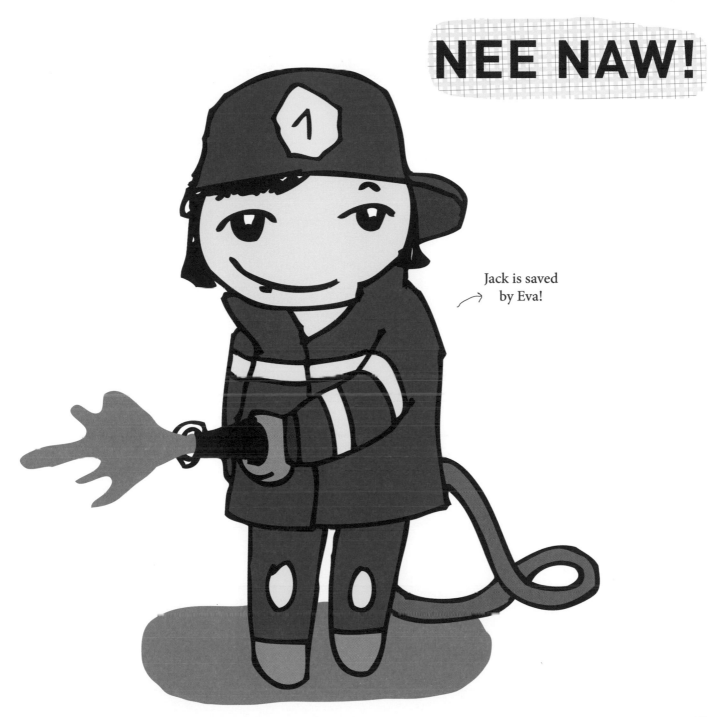

NEE NAW!

Jack is saved by Eva!

ROCK & ROLL

Jack's Mum and Dad are very good at dancing. Sometimes they do the tango.
Then they look at each other as if they're angry. Jack prefers watching them dance
to rock and roll most. Then Mum's skirt swirls around so fast that Jack can feel
the air brush across his cheeks. And sometimes Jack gets to dance along.

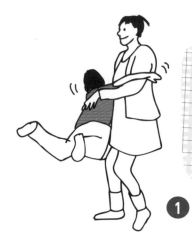

Jack stands a fair distance from Mum and runs toward her with outstretched arms. Mum grabs him under his arms and twirls him around.

1

2

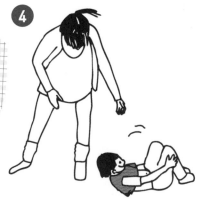

Next she whirls him around her hip and lets go of one hand. She uses her free hand to hook the back of Jack's knees against the other side of her back. They dance like this around the room for a few minutes.

3

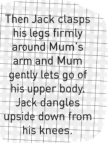

Then Jack clasps his legs firmly around Mum's arm and Mum gently lets go of his upper body. Jack dangles upside down from his knees.

4

He places his hands on the floor, looks at his stomach and rolls in a little ball to his feet. 'Ta da!'

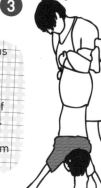

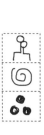

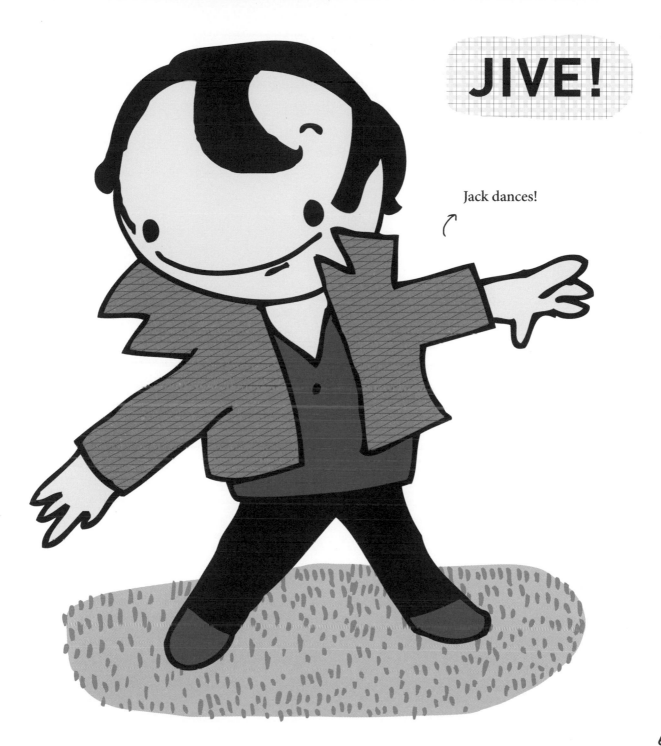

JIVE!

Jack dances!

THE FLYING MACHINE

When he grows up, Jack wants to be a pilot.
From his garden, he waves at all the planes. 'Woohoo!'

Outside, he practises flying with Mum and Dad. Jack lies on the ground and Mum and Dad pick him up by his ankles and wrists. They rock him gently backward and forward, each time aiming a little higher.

Dad counts: 'One, two, three!' And wahey! Jack is standing on their shoulders.

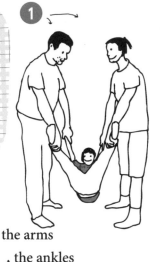

the arms
the ankles

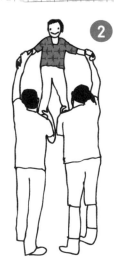

This trick is a little scary but exciting too. Ideally, Mum and Dad should practise with a jumper first. The arms are Jack's arms and the lower corners of the jumper are his ankles. They swing the jumper really high. On the count of three, they each turn the shoulder of the hand that holds the ankle toward each other. In this way, they place Jack's feet on their shoulders, holding him firmly until he is upright and towers above everyone else.

close-up

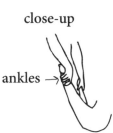

ankles →

Would you like to be placed on the ground in the same way, straight down with your bottom facing away?

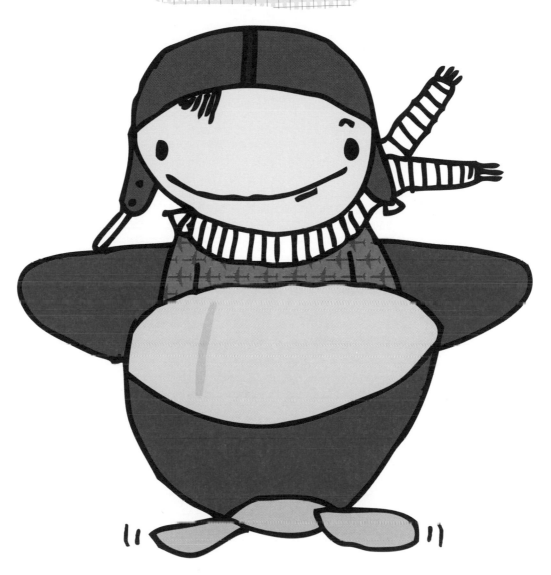

AND NOW... SHOWTIME

Finally, the time has come: the Christmas tree is shimmering with decorations and the whole house smells of turkey. Tonight, the entire family is coming to dinner. These past few weeks, Jack and Dad have been hard at work practising their acrobatic show. Jack's sister has chosen some nice music to accompany their act. Mum has found some costumes. Rabbit will be placed on top of the highest pyramid. And Jack's brother has promised to applaud loudly. Ready? Let's begin!

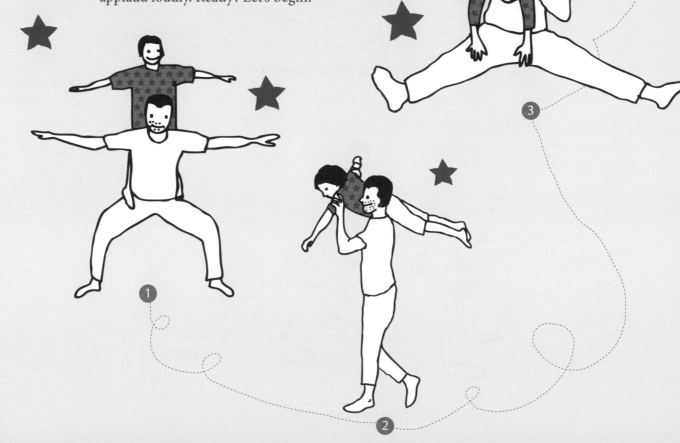

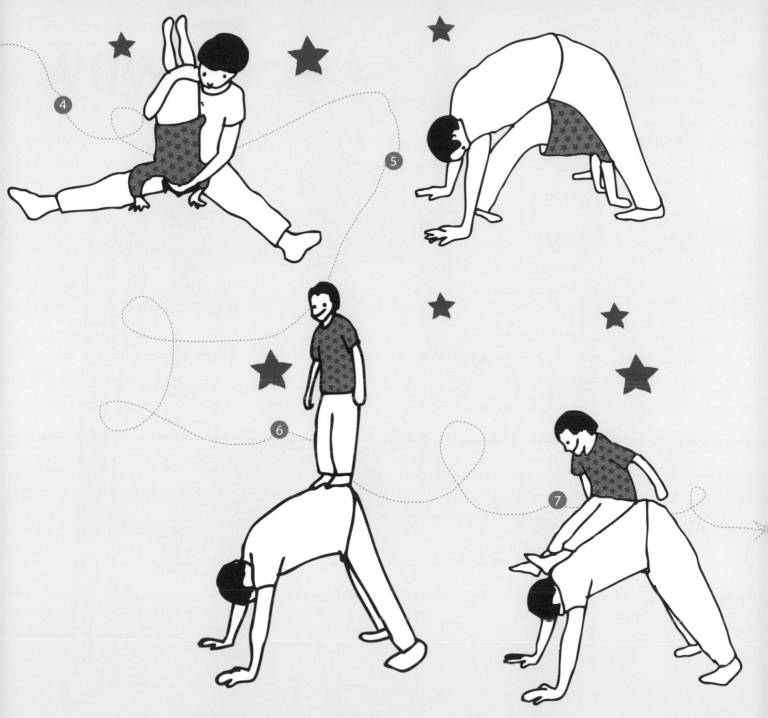

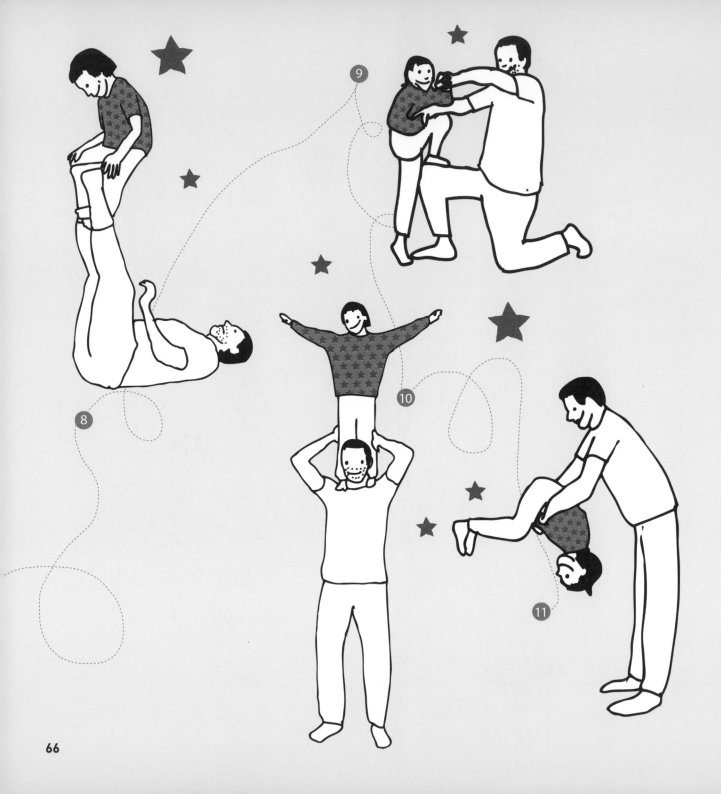

Jack and Dad take a deep bow and his sister turns off the music.
Grandad jumps up from the table and applauds loudly. Grandma
shouts 'Bravo!' and Mum looks really proud.
'You're a true acrobat!' Auntie shouts. Jack is sure of it –
this has been the best Christmas ever.

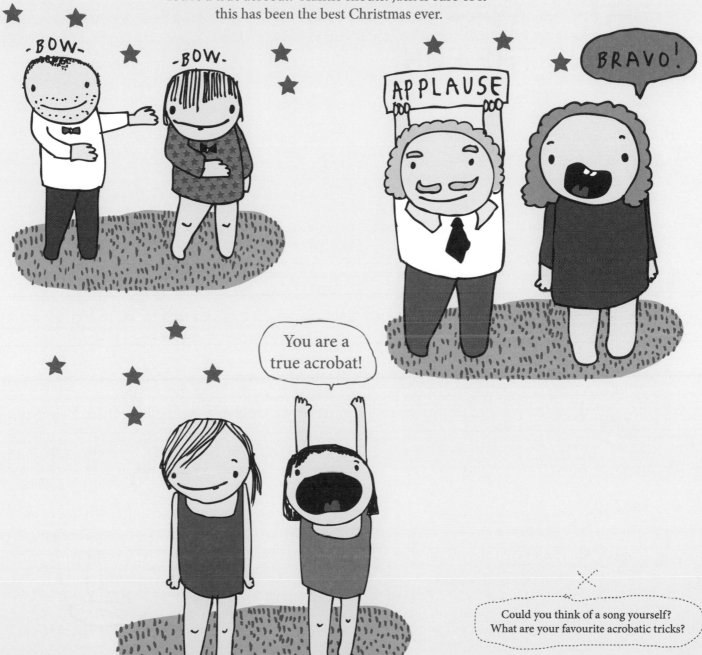

THE THEORY BEHIND THE FUN

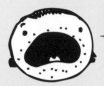

'Circomotorics is all about pushing boundaries, gaining trust and cuddling. It's all about intense contact with your child.'

LUCAS'S DAD

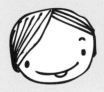

'I like learning new things and playing together with my mum and dad.'

EMMA, four years old

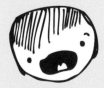

'The pyramids are fun and exciting to do.'

ELLE, five years old

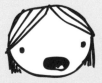

'Your child trains their motor skills in a subtle way, without being forced. It's much more fun than the obligatory gymnastics.'

RIK'S MUM

The acrobatics in this book stem from the circus, and the practice games from Sherborne's developmental movement. Rika Taeymans developed this mixture of circus and movement philosophy in the nineties and christened it 'circomotorics'. The skills needed to perform acrobatics tricks safely and without fear are taught in a playful environment through practise games. In addition to physical skills and improved self-awareness, the exercises are a means of providing emotional stimulation through relationship games.

According to Veronica Sherborne, children have two very basic needs – they need to feel at home in their own bodies and they need to be able to form relationships.

acrobatics   practice games

AT HOME IN YOUR BODY

Children become aware of their arms, legs and head first. It's not until much later that they learn they have an upper body, a centre if you will, that connects everything. Unsurprisingly, the first portraits from toddlers are often 'head footers'.

Three important skills in a child's motor development are: learning how to tuck themselves into a tight ball around their core, and tensing and relaxing the upper body. The exercises in this book are therefore constructed around the ability to form a ball, tense the body like a board and relax into free flow. Results are best when all three are practised randomly.

A child needs to be aware of his own body, of how strong he is and what he can do. This way, he learns to trust himself and gauge what he can and what he can and can't do. A child can only be comfortable in his own body when he *knows* his own body.

When a child takes a significant step in the development of his motor skills, he also takes a mental leap and something fundamental changes in his perception of the world. A child who, for example, after lots of practice, gets over his fear of standing on dad's shoulders, will experience that as a real victory.

BALLS AND SOMERSAULTS

Learning to tuck himself into a little ball is an important and challenging step for your child. From an early age, children have the inherent instinct to stretch their arms and legs when they fall. It's an incorrect reflex. Tucking yourself around your centre is therefore an important skill in learning how to fall safely.

The practice games in this book start with the sideways roll, as in the exercise with the strands of spaghetti (page 56). This way of rolling is the easiest. But it's also important to learn how to tumble forward or backward over head and shoulders.

Lying on their backs, young children (aged three and four) often find it difficult to touch their noses to their knees. Their head seems to be too heavy. Five-year-olds learn how to do this a lot quicker. With the forward tumble, children often find it hard to tuck their heads in and remain in a tight ball to the end.

In the exercise with the rocking chair (page 50) you can guide the forward roll with your hands and teach your child how to position his neck by letting him tumble over your shoulder and into the rocking chair. You can also practise the backward tumble in the rocking chair by letting your child roll out of the chair.

The ultimate test to determine whether or not your child is aware of his centre, is to lift him up in a ball and see of he remains tucked in a ball even when in mid-air, as the ravioli (page 56) or the snowman (page 14). Once your child can form a ball, he's ready for the proper somersaults.

BOARDS AND PYRAMIDS

In order to build pyramids, you need to be strong and feel at ease in your own body. Relaxing the upper body (both stomach and back) with the hips and shoulders as important hinges can be tricky for some children. It takes a while for them to master this skill and to not let their bellies flop. 'Practice makes perfect' is the message here. By playing the practice games carrying the symbol of a board, children learn to adopt the right kind of tension. It shows them how stable and strong they can be.

Pyramids can be scary sometimes, in which case an assistant can be a great help. You don't assist by holding hands, but by being near and at the ready. And if you do prefer to physically support your child, it's much better to hold him by his hips rather than his hands.

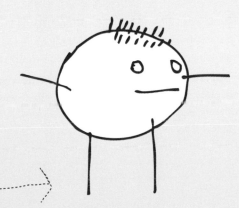

FREE FLOW AND WHIRL

Free flow movements are movements that are difficult to stop. It can be immensely liberating to be swung and twirled around. But not every child is capable of being uninhibited and surrendering to another person. Free flow games teach children to relax their upper bodies and limbs. They learn how to let go of physical and mental control and lose their fear of fast movements. When they do these types of exercises often, they'll be less afraid to swing on a trapeze or whizz down a hill on a sledge later on in life.

RELATIONSHIP GAMES

Relationship games are fun and instructive. Children learn about various relationship forms in a playful way. They learn how to stand up for themselves, to care for someone and to collaborate with another. As a parent, by giving positive encouragement, you create a secure and safe environment in which your child can explore and learn on their own. By learning how to deal with relationships playfully in a secure environment, your child will be more adept in the outside world.

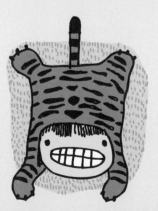

In her teachings, Veronica Sherborne works with three kinds of relationships: **the 'with relationships', the 'against relationships' and the 'together relationships'.**

In the 'against' games, a child learns to be strong, to stand up for what he wants and to control his strength. These games only succeed if you really commit to them and don't give up. Grandma's gift that doesn't want to be opened yet is a good example (page 18). The child needs to concentrate and learns to fight for what he wants. Active children will have a lot of fun with this game. The more reserved children will first need to develop a level of trust within themselves and their partner.

Most children like resistance games involving pulling and pushing. In the positions described they will often feel that their parent is actually pushing quite hard, but that they can still win. This will make them feel good, strong and self-confident. The tiger rug (page 30) is a good example of this. There's obviously the agreement that you don't hurt each other, and tickling is also a no-go. Resistance games are not contests, but rather a fun and challenging game between two partners.

It's very important not to pull or push hard and erratically. Start with a gentle application of force. Show your child clearly the direction in which he can resist. Then you can gradually increase the pressure. As the parent, you follow the tempo of your child. Obviously it's fun to let children win, but make them work for it – it's even more fun when they experience a real sense of having earned it. And it always feels good to let off some steam.

The 'with' games teach a child to care for someone else, and to relax when being looked after by that person. Children learn the meaning of being nice in a very physical and, for them, comprehensible way. These exercises repeatedly involve one active partner and one passive, relaxed partner. Carefully unwrapping a gift illustrates this principle well (page 18). The gift relaxes every muscle and lets himself be manipulated and moved. This way, you learn alternately to care for and trust one another.

Children are often more comfortable with one of the two relationships, but as yet haven't found the right balance. Some children are as stubborn as mules and are really adept at playing the 'against' games, although they might have a harder time relaxing and caring for a brother or sister. Other children are very sweet and mild-mannered, but are uncomfortable with being determined and really going after something. They give in more easily and can in the 'against' games learn how to persevere and defend themselves better. When there's a balance between these polar opposites, you're ready to synchronise and collaborate.

'Together' games stimulate collaboration. It's only possible for you to build a pyramid if you both feel strong and trust each other. It also demands a lot of concentration and endurance.

Can't picture it yet? Imagine two adults sitting back to back. They can work together in this position. One person can lean against his partner's back and be rocked. But they can also work against each other and push against each other to see who can push the other furthest. In collaboration, they can ultimately try to stand together by pushing shoulders and back together and not relinquishing for one second. Trust and synchronisation are needed for this.

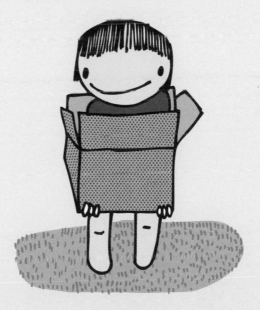

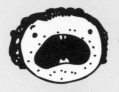

'What a child can do in cooperation today, he will do alone tomorrow.'

VYGOTSKY
(Russian psychologist)

Where the possibility arises, it's fun to change roles in every game and have parent and child alternate, thus allowing both to take the initiative at some point. By attributing the fun role of boss to your child, he feels that you trust him. As a parent, you get the chance to be less demanding and dictatorial – you listen to your child and respond to his signals. By venturing to his level – to roll, lie or sit down – he becomes larger than you. This gives your child the opportunity to view you from a different perspective than normal – a magical thing for children. Eye contact becomes a lot easier and more pleasant and children feel more your equal. But parents gain from this 'shrinking' experience as well – moving around on the floor makes you more flexible and – perhaps after a period of stiffness – you go through life with a great deal more agility.

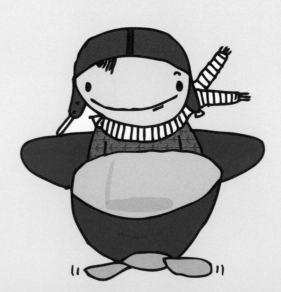

VERONICA SHERBORNE

Veronica Sherborne (UK) was a teacher of physical education, a physiotherapist and mother of three children. Through contact with her pupils and her own children, she realised the importance of physical contact in the development of a child. Babies and children learn a tremendous amount about themselves by being physically carried and supported in the first years of their lives. Children are not yet verbal at that stage and rely to a great extent on the physical and non-verbal. Physical and eye contact allow children to develop self-awareness and their boundaries, and it makes them more confident in their own bodies. Moving together and playing games is incredibly important to both parent and child from his first year. It is a great way to get to know each other, to react to each other and become attuned to one another. Once this becomes a positive action–reaction game, the child will gain all the self-confidence he needs to build relationships in the outside world.

Sherborne worked with children who suffered from emotional and behavioural problems such as ADHD and autism. At a later stage in her career, she worked with adults with psychological problems as well. Her book, *Developmental Movement for Children*, is a record of twenty-six years of experience with people with learning difficulties and physical disabilities. She noticed that parents gave less attention to children with a condition that manifested itself at an early age because these children were slower and responded less to signals and games. Their condition, however, meant they needed more stimulation and attention. This is why she developed a method that makes people aware of their own bodies and strengths through simple games.

Sherborne's games allow anyone to move together in a natural and spontaneous way. Her play encourages children to be very strong and powerful on the one hand, and kind and supportive on the other, all in a non-verbal, pleasant way. Feeling comfortable in your own body and knowing its possibilities is crucial to the development of a positive self-image and a healthy dose of self-confidence.

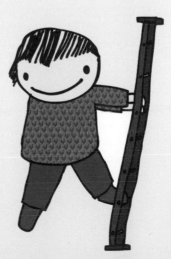

THANK YOU

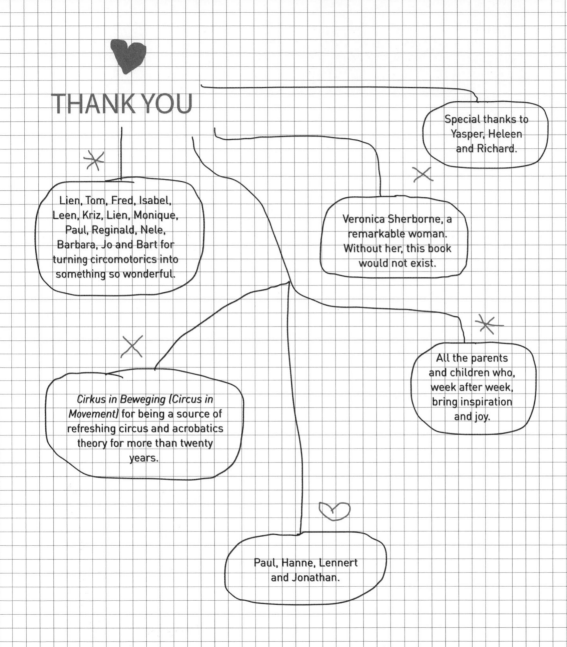

Special thanks to Yasper, Heleen and Richard.

Lien, Tom, Fred, Isabel, Leen, Kriz, Lien, Monique, Paul, Reginald, Nele, Barbara, Jo and Bart for turning circomotorics into something so wonderful.

Veronica Sherborne, a remarkable woman. Without her, this book would not exist.

Cirkus in Beweging (Circus in Movement) for being a source of refreshing circus and acrobatics theory for more than twenty years.

All the parents and children who, week after week, bring inspiration and joy.

Paul, Hanne, Lennert and Jonathan.

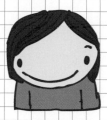

RIKA TAEYMANS

In 1993, Rika founded *Cirkus in Beweging (Circus in Movement)*, the very first Flemish circus school. It's where she developed circomotorics, a playful form of exercise based on a mixture of acrobatics and Veronica Sherborne's developmental movement learning. Circomotorics is all about having fun and maintaining the physical contact between parents and kids. For more than twenty years, Rika has been getting up very early every Saturday morning to give more than one hundred children lessons in making somersaults and building pyramids with their dads, mums, grandmothers or grandfathers.

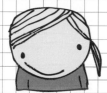

LAURA VAN BOUCHOUT

As a child Laura preferred walking on her hands to walking on her feet. She was one of Rika's first pupils and loved swinging on the trapeze. After ten years of practice, she became Rika's colleague in circomotorics. Nowadays, she prefers writing to swinging on the trapeze. Together with Rika, she decided to write down some of the exercises so that many more children would have the chance to enjoy these exciting games. Laura bakes pancakes every Saturday morning.

EMMA THYSSEN

Emma hasn't as yet stood on top of a pyramid, but she can execute a perfect handstand. She is very good at drawing and has created a lot of beautiful books. When Emma draws, the tip of her tongue sneaks out of the corner of her mouth. Her favourite colour is red with pink stripes. On Saturday mornings she loves to lie in and she drinks large mugs of green tea.

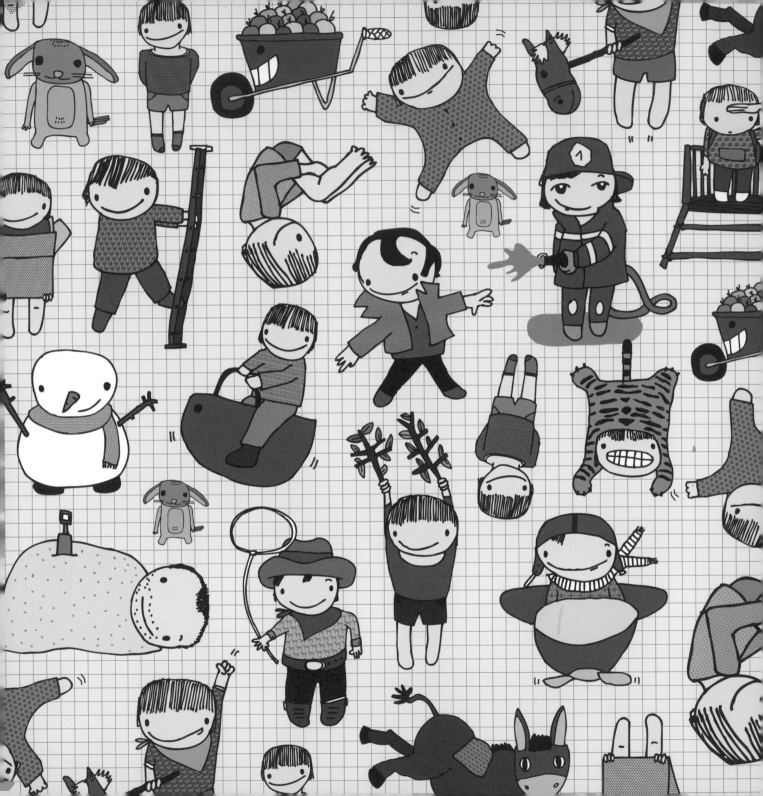